Ga[...] is:
an introduction

Fourth Edition

For Elsevier:

This book is dedicated to:
Wendy
Jim and Maeve
Sally, Garrie, Samuel and Gregory
Robert and Mia
Tracey, Jermaine and Will

Publisher: Heidi Harrison
Associate Editor: Siobhan Campbell
Production Manager: Elouise Ball
Design: Andy Chapman
Illustrator: Robert Britton
Illustration Buyer: Merlyn Harvey

Gait Analysis:
An introduction
FOURTH EDITION

Michael W. Whittle BSc, MB, BS, MSc, PhD
Walter M. Cline Chair of Excellence in Rehabilitation Technology
The University of Tennessee at Chattanooga
Chattanooga, Tennessee, USA

and

Director
H. Carey Hanlin Motion Analysis Laboratory
The University of Tennessee at Chattanooga
Chattanooga, Tennessee, USA

formerly

Acting Director
Oxford Orthopaedic Engineering Centre
University of Oxford
Oxford, UK

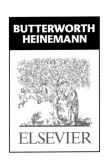

BUTTERWORTH
HEINEMANN

ELSEVIER

EDINBURGH   LONDON   NEW YORK   OXFORD   PHILADELPHIA   ST LOUIS   SYDNEY   TORONTO 2007

BUTTERWORTH
HEINEMANN
ELSEVIER

An imprint of Elsevier Limited
First published 1990
Second edition 1996
Reprinted 1997
Third edition 2002
Reprinted 2003 (twice), 2004, 2005
Fourth edition 2007
Reprinted 2008

ISBN: 9 780 7506 8883 3

British Library Cataloguing in Publication Data
A catalogue record for this book is available from the British Library.

Library of Congress Cataloging in Publication Data
A catalog record for this book is available from the Library of Congress.

Note

Neither the Publisher nor the Authors assume any responsibility for any loss or injury and/or damage to persons or property arising out of or related to any use of the material contained in this book. It is the responsibility of the treating practitioner, relying on independent expertise and knowledge of the patient, to determine the best treatment and method of application for the patient.

Printed in China

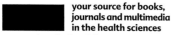
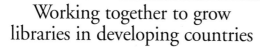

Contents

Acknowledgments   vii
Preface to fourth edition   ix
Preface to first edition   xi

1   Basic sciences   1
Anatomy   1
Physiology   19
Biomechanics   31
References and suggestions for further reading   45

2   Normal gait   47
Walking and gait   47
History   48
Terminology used in gait analysis   52
Outline of the gait cycle   57
The gait cycle in detail   64
Ground reaction forces   80
Support moment   84
Energy consumption   84
Optimization of energy usage   87
Starting and stopping   92
Other varieties of gait   93
Gait in the young   94
Gait in the elderly   96
References and suggestions for further reading   98

3   Pathological and other abnormal gaits   101
Specific gait abnormalities   102
Walking aids   122
Amputee gait   129
Treadmill gait   133
Common pathologies affecting gait   134
References and suggestions for further reading   135

4   Methods of gait analysis   137
Visual gait analysis   137
General gait parameters   143
Timing the gait cycle   146
Direct motion measurement systems   148
Electrogoniometers   149
Pressure beneath the foot   152
Electromyography   154
Energy consumption   157

Accelerometers   159
Gyroscopes   160
Force platforms   160
Kinematic systems   165
Combined kinetic/kinematic systems   172
References and suggestions for further reading   174

5   Applications of gait analysis   177
Clinical gait assessment   178
Conditions benefiting from gait assessment   187
Future developments   191
Conclusion   192
References and suggestions for further reading   192

6   Gait assessment in cerebral palsy   195
Basic physiology of movement   195
The causes of cerebral palsy   196
Spastic hemiplegia   197
Spastic diplegia   199
Other varieties of cerebral palsy   200
Crouch gait   201
Spasticity   202
Lever arm dysfunction   203
Gait patterns in cerebral palsy   204
Gait assessment   209
Overview of treatment   214
Summary   216
References and suggestions for further reading   217

7   Gait analysis data on CD-ROM   219
Computer requirements   219
Running the CD   219
Contents of the CD   220
How to use the Polygon viewer   220
Notes   222
Acknowledgments   222
Appendices   223
   1. Normal ranges for gait parameters   223
   2. Conversions between measurement units   225
   3. Sources of further information   229

Glossary   233
Index   243

Acknowledgments

I would particularly like to thank my wife, Wendy, for her encouragement, support and tolerance while I have been preparing this book. Particular thanks are also due to Karen Hood, Jeannette Beach and Locke Davis, who work with me in the gait laboratory and have taught me so much about clinical gait analysis. The CD-ROM which accompanies this book contains data generously supplied by Nancy Denniston and her colleagues at the Children's Hospital, Denver, and some text written by Chris Kirtley. The Polygon computer program, used to prepare the interactive multimedia presentation of gait, was provided through the generosity of Vicon Peak Ltd. Three other groups have also contributed in different ways to this book: my faculty colleagues, the students I teach and the patients we have seen in the laboratory. I would finally like to thank the administrators of The University of Tennessee at Chattanooga for their support.

Preface
to fourth edition

Gait analysis is the systematic study of human walking, using the eye and brain of experienced observers, augmented by instrumentation for measuring body movements, body mechanics and the activity of the muscles. In individuals with conditions affecting their ability to walk, gait analysis may be used to make detailed diagnoses and to plan optimal treatment.

Over the past few years, gait analysis has 'come of age' and in a number of centers it is now used routinely to provide the best possible care for certain groups of patients, most notably those with cerebral palsy. Since the benefits of this approach have been well established, it is to be hoped that its usage will continue to spread, so that many more will benefit from the better treatment decisions which can be made when gait analysis is used.

I am happy to believe that the first three editions of this book have contributed to this process, by providing a text which does not require a high level of academic learning to be understood. I have heard from people all over the world that they have found the book useful and this I find very gratifying.

The next stage in the evolution of gait analysis will hopefully involve improvements in the ease and speed with which gait data can be collected and interpreted, and decreases in the cost of the equipment and the skill level needed to use it. Significant strides have been made in all these aspects since the third edition of the book was published in 2002 but there is clearly still room for improvement.

The inclusion of a CD-ROM with 'real' gait data with this book will, it is hoped, provide the reader with a better opportunity to get a feel for this fascinating subject.

Michael W. Whittle
2007

Preface
to first edition

Gait analysis is the systematic study of human walking. It is often helpful in the medical management of those diseases which affect the locomotor system. Over the past few years, there has been an increasing interest in the subject, particularly among practitioners and students of physical therapy, bio-engineering, neurology and rehabilitation. Most previous books on the subject have been written for specialists and are thus unsuitable for the student or general reader. I have attempted to write an introductory textbook, with the aim of providing the reader with a solid grounding in the subject but without assuming a particular background or level of prior knowledge.

Chapter 1 is devoted to the basic sciences underlying gait analysis – anatomy, physiology and biomechanics. It is intended to give the reader who is new to these subjects the minimum required to make sense of gait analysis. It should also provide a refresher course for those who have once had such knowledge but forgotten it, as well as being a convenient source of reference material. Chapters 2 and 3 deal with normal gait and pathological gait respectively, showing the remarkable efficiency of the normal walking process and the various ways in which it may be affected by disease. Chapter 4 is devoted to methods of measurement, pointing out that gait analysis does not have to be difficult or expensive but that the more complicated systems provide detailed information which cannot be obtained in any other way. The final chapter, Chapter 5, deals with the applications of gait analysis. This is the area in which the most progress is to be anticipated in the future. The literature of the field is heavily biased towards research rather than clinical application but the value of the methodology is gradually coming to be realized in a number of clinical conditions.

I deliberately avoided giving references to theses and conference proceedings, since these may be difficult to find. Chapter 1 contains no references at all, as everything in it should be easy to find in standard textbooks. I have restricted the number of references quoted in the remainder of the book, not through ignorance or laziness but rather in an attempt to identify only the most important references on particular topics. These will in turn lead on to other references, should the reader wish to study that topic in greater detail. Those not familiar with it should ask their librarian about the Science Citation Index, which uses key references from the past to identify more recent publications in the same field.

I have used the Système International (SI) units throughout this book. I make no apology for this – everyone working in this field should be using the measurement units of science, rather than those of the grocery store! However, conversions are given in Appendix 2.

Since the origins of this book are international, it is hoped that it will appeal to an international readership. It was written during my last few months at the University of Oxford, UK, and my first few months at the University of Tennessee at Chattanooga, in the USA. It draws on reference material from both sides of the Atlantic and parts of it were written on journeys across that ocean!

Michael W. Whittle
Chattanooga, Tennessee
May 1990

Basic sciences

I

All voluntary movement, including walking, results from a complicated process involving the brain, spinal cord, peripheral nerves, muscles, bones and joints. Before considering in detail the process of walking, what can go wrong with it and how it can be studied, it is necessary to have a basic understanding of three scientific disciplines: anatomy, physiology and biomechanics. It is hoped that this chapter will provide the rudiments of these subjects for those not already familiar with them, will review the topic for those who are, and will also provide a convenient source of reference material.

ANATOMY

It is not the intention of this book to teach in detail the anatomy of the locomotor system, which is well covered in several other books (e.g. Palastanga *et al.*, 1989). The notes which follow give only an outline of the subject, but one which should be sufficient for an understanding of gait analysis. The anatomical names for the different parts of the body vary somewhat from one textbook to another; as far as possible the most common name has been used. The section starts by describing some basic anatomical terms and then goes on to describe the bones, joints, muscles and nervous system. Although the arteries and veins are essential to the functioning of the locomotor system, they will not be described here since they generally affect gait only indirectly, through their role in providing oxygen and nutrients for the nerves and muscles and removing waste products.

Basic anatomical terms

The anatomical terms describing the relationships between different parts of the body are based on the *anatomical position*, in which a person is standing upright, with the feet together and the arms by the sides of the body, with the palms forward. This position, together with the reference planes and the terms describing relationships between different parts of the body, is illustrated in Fig. 1.1.

Six terms are used to describe directions, with relation to the center of the body. These are best defined by example:

1. The umbilicus is *anterior*
2. The buttocks are *posterior*
3. The head is *superior*
4. The feet are *inferior*
5. *Left* is self-evident
6. So is *right*.

The anterior surface of the body is *ventral* and the posterior surface is *dorsal*. The word *dorsum* is used for both the back of the hand and the upper surface

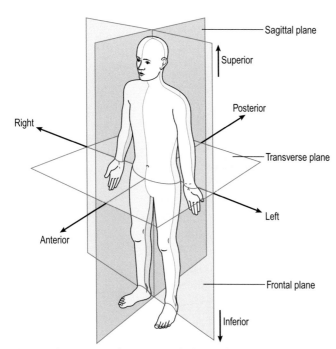

Right

Anterior

Sagittal plane

Superior

Posterior

Transverse plane

Left

Frontal plane

Inferior

Fig. 1.1 The anatomical position, with three reference planes and six fundamental directions.

of the foot. The terms *cephalad* (towards the head) and *caudad* (towards the 'tail') are sometimes used in place of superior and inferior.

Within a single part of the body, six additional terms are used to describe relationships:

1. *Medial* means towards the midline of the body: the big toe is on the medial side of the foot
2. *Lateral* means away from the midline of the body: the little toe is on the lateral side of the foot
3. *Proximal* means towards the rest of the body: the shoulder is the proximal part of the arm
4. *Distal* means away from the rest of the body: the fingers are the distal part of the hand
5. *Superficial* structures are close to the surface
6. *Deep* structures are far from the surface.

The motion of the limbs is described using reference planes:

1. A *sagittal* plane is any plane which divides part of the body into right and left portions; the *median* plane is the midline sagittal plane, which divides the whole body into right and left halves
2. A *frontal* plane divides a body part into front and back portions
3. A *transverse* plane divides a body part into upper and lower portions.

The term *coronal plane* is equivalent to frontal plane and the transverse plane may also be called the *horizontal plane*, although it is only horizontal when in the standing position.

Most joints can only move in one or two of these three planes. The directions of these motions for the hip and knee are shown in Fig. 1.2 and for the ankle and foot in Fig. 1.3. The possible movements are as follows:

1. *Flexion* and *extension* take place in the sagittal plane; in the ankle these movements are called *dorsiflexion* and *plantarflexion*, respectively
2. *Abduction* and *adduction* take place in the frontal plane
3. *Internal* and *external* rotation take place in the transverse plane; they are also called *medial* and *lateral* rotation respectively, the term referring to the motion of the anterior surface.

Other terms which are used to describe the motions of the joints or body segments are:

1. *Varus* and *valgus*, which describe an angulation of a joint towards or away from the midline, respectively; knock knees are in valgus, bow legs are in varus

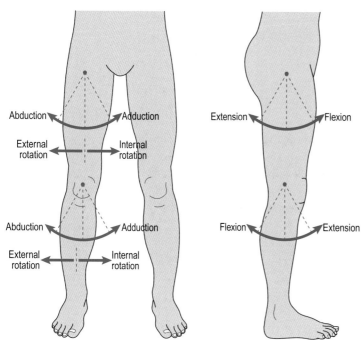

Fig. 1.2 Movements about the hip joint (above) and knee joint (below).

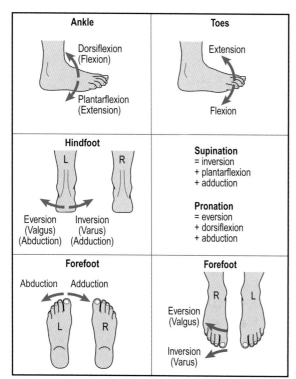

Fig. 1.3 Movements of the ankle, toes, hindfoot and forefoot.

2. *Pronation* and *supination*, which are rotations about the long axis of the forearm or foot; pronation of both hands brings the thumbs together, supination brings the little fingers together (aide-memoire: you can hold *soup* in your hands if the palms are upwards)
3. *Inversion* of the feet brings the soles together; *eversion* causes the soles to point away from the midline.

Terminology in the foot is often confusing and lacking in standardization. This book has adopted what is probably the commonest convention (Fig. 1.3), in which the term *pronation* is used for a combined movement which consists primarily of eversion but also includes some dorsiflexion and forefoot abduction. Similarly, supination is primarily inversion, but also includes some plantarflexion and forefoot adduction. These movements represent a 'twisting' of the forefoot, relative to the hindfoot. However, some authorities regard pronation and supination as the basic movements and eversion and inversion as the combined movements.

Bones

It could be argued that almost every bone in the body takes part in walking. However, from a practical point of view, it is generally only necessary to consider the bones of the pelvis and legs. These are shown in Fig. 1.4.

The *pelvis* is formed from the sacrum, the coccyx and the two innominate bones. The *sacrum* consists of the five sacral vertebrae, fused together. The *coccyx* is the vestigial 'tail', made of three to five rudimentary vertebrae. The *innominate bone* on each side is formed by the fusion of three bones: the *ilium, ischium* and *pubis*. The only real movement between the bones of the pelvis occurs at the sacroiliac joint and this movement is generally very small in adults. It is thus reasonable, for the purposes of gait analysis, to regard the pelvis as being a single rigid structure. The superior surface of the sacrum articulates with the fifth lumbar vertebra of the spine. On each side of the lower part of the pelvis is the acetabulum, which is the proximal part of the hip joint, being the socket into which the head of the femur fits.

The *femur* is the longest bone in the body. The spherical femoral head articulates with the pelvic acetabulum to form the hip joint. The neck of the femur runs downwards and laterally from the femoral head to meet the shaft of the bone, which continues downwards to the knee joint. At the junction of the neck and the shaft are two bony protuberances, where a number of muscles are inserted – the greater trochanter laterally, which can be felt beneath the skin, and the lesser trochanter medially. The bone widens at its lower end to form the medial and lateral condyles. These form the proximal part of the knee joint and have a groove between them anteriorly, which articulates with the patella.

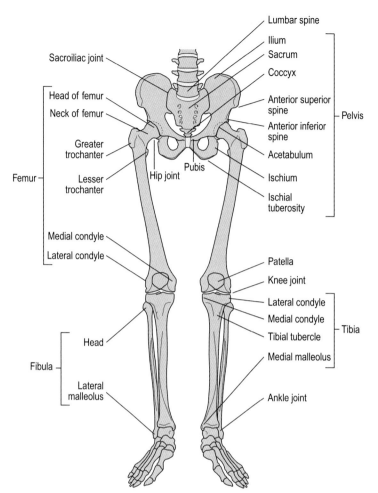

Fig. 1.4 Bones and joints of the lower limbs.

The *patella* or kneecap is a sesamoid bone; that is to say, it is embedded within a tendon, in this case the massive quadriceps tendon, which below the patella is known as the patellar tendon. The anterior surface of the patella is subcutaneous (immediately below the skin); its posterior surface articulates with the anterior surface of the lower end of the femur to form the patellofemoral joint. The patella has an important mechanical function, which is to displace the quadriceps tendon forwards, thereby improving its leverage.

The *tibia* extends from the knee joint to the ankle joint. Its upper end is broadened into medial and lateral condyles, with an almost flat upper surface which articulates with the femur. The tibial tubercle is a small bony prominence on the front of the tibia, where the patellar tendon is inserted. The anterior surface of the tibia is subcutaneous. The lower end of the tibia forms the upper and medial surfaces of the ankle joint, with a subcutaneous medial projection called the medial malleolus.

The *fibula* is next to the tibia on its lateral side. For most of its length it is a fairly slim bone, although it is broadened at both ends, the upper end being known as the head. The broadened lower end forms the lateral part of the ankle joint, with a subcutaneous lateral projection known as the lateral malleolus. The tibia and fibula are in contact with each other at their upper and lower ends, as the tibiofibular joints. Movements at these joints are very small and will not be considered further. A layer of fibrous tissue, known as the interosseous membrane, lies between the bones.

The foot is a very complicated structure (Fig. 1.5), which is best thought of as being in three parts:

1. The *hindfoot*, which consists of two bones, one on top of the other
2. The *midfoot*, which consists of five bones, packed closely together
3. The *forefoot*, which consists of the five metatarsals and the toes.

The *talus* or astragalus is the upper of the two bones in the hindfoot. Its superior surface forms the ankle joint, articulating above and medially with the tibia and laterally with the fibula. Below, the talus articulates with the calcaneus through the subtalar joint. It articulates anteriorly with the most medial and superior of the midfoot bones – the navicular.

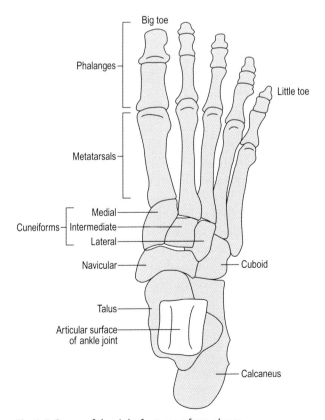

Fig. 1.5 Bones of the right foot, seen from above.

The *calcaneus* or os calcis lies below the talus and articulates with it through the subtalar joint. Its lower surface transmits the body weight to the ground through a thick layer of fat, fibrous tissue and skin – the heelpad. The anterior surface articulates with the most lateral and inferior of the midfoot bones – the cuboid.

The midfoot consists of five bones:

1. The *navicular*, which is medial and superior
2. The *cuboid*, which is lateral and inferior
3. Three *cuneiform* bones (medial, intermediate and lateral), which lie in a row, distal to the navicular.

The five *metatarsals* lie roughly parallel to each other, the lateral two articulating with the cuboid and the medial three with the three cuneiform bones.

The *phalanges* are the bones of the toes; there are two in the big toe and three in each of the other toes. The big toe is also called the great toe or *hallux*.

Joints and ligaments

A joint occurs where one bone is in contact with another. From a practical point of view, they can be divided into synovial joints, in which significant movement can take place, and the various other types of joint in which only small movements can occur. Since gait analysis is normally only concerned with fairly large movements, the description which follows deals only with synovial joints. In a *synovial joint*, the bone ends are covered in *cartilage* and the joint is surrounded by a *synovial capsule*, which secretes the lubricant *synovial fluid*. Most joints are stabilized by *ligaments*, which are bands of relatively inelastic fibrous tissue connecting one bone to another. *Fascia* is a special type of ligament, being a continuous sheet of fibrous tissue.

The *hip* joint is the only true ball-and-socket joint in the body, the ball being the head of the femur and the socket the acetabulum of the pelvis. Extremes of movement are prevented by a number of ligaments running between the pelvis and the femur, by a capsule surrounding the joint and by a small ligament – the ligamentum teres – which joins the center of the head of the femur to the center of the acetabulum. The joint is capable of flexion, extension, abduction, adduction, internal and external rotation (Fig. 1.2).

The *knee* joint consists of the medial and lateral condyles of the femur, above, and the corresponding condyles of the tibia, below. The articular surfaces on the medial and lateral sides are separate, making the knee joint, in effect, two joints, side by side. The femoral condyles are curved both from front to back and from side to side, whereas the tibial condyles are almost flat. The 'gap' this would leave around the point of contact is filled, on each side, by a 'meniscus', commonly called a 'cartilage', which acts to spread the load and reduce the pressure at the point of contact.

The motion of the joint is controlled by five ligaments which, between them, exert very close control over the movements of the knee:

1. The medial collateral ligament (MCL), which prevents the medial side of the joint from opening up (i.e. it opposes abduction or valgus)
2. The lateral collateral ligament (LCL) similarly opposes adduction or varus
3. The posterior joint capsule, which prevents hyperextension (excessive extension) of the joint
4. The anterior cruciate ligament (ACL), in the center of the joint, between the condyles; it is attached to the tibia anteriorly and the femur posteriorly. It prevents the tibia from moving forwards relative to the femur and helps to prevent excessive rotation
5. The posterior cruciate ligament (PCL), also in the center of the joint, is attached to the tibia posteriorly and the femur anteriorly and prevents the tibia from moving backwards relative to the femur and also helps to limit rotation.

The anterior and posterior cruciate ligaments are named for the positions in which they are attached to the tibia. They appear to act together as what engineers call a 'four-bar linkage', which imposes a combination of sliding and rolling on the joint and moves the contact point forwards as the joint extends and backwards as it flexes. This means that the axis about which the joint flexes and extends is not fixed, but changes with the angle of flexion or extension. Pollo *et al.* (2003) challenged this description, saying that it only occurs in the unloaded knee and that during walking, the tibia moves backwards relative to the femur as the knee flexes.

In the normal individual, the motions of the knee are flexion and extension, with a small amount of internal and external rotation. Significant amounts of abduction and adduction are only seen in damaged knees. As the knee comes to full extension, there is an external rotation of a few degrees: the so-called automatic rotation or 'screw-home' mechanism.

The *patellofemoral* joint lies between the posterior surface of the patella and the anterior surface of the femur. The articular surface consists of a shallow V-shaped ridge on the patella, which fits into a shallow groove between the medial and lateral condyles. The principal movement is the patella gliding up and down in this groove, during extension and flexion of the knee, respectively. This causes different areas of the patella to come into contact with different parts of the joint surfaces of the femur. There is also some medial–lateral movement of the patella.

The *ankle* or talocrural joint has three surfaces: upper, medial and lateral. The upper surface is the main articulation of the joint; it is cylindrical and formed by the tibia above and the talus below. The medial joint surface is between the talus and the inner aspect of the medial malleolus of the tibia.

Correspondingly, the lateral joint surface is between the talus and the inner surface of the lateral malleolus of the fibula.

The major ligaments of the ankle joint are those between the tibia and the fibula, preventing these two bones from moving apart, and the collateral ligaments on both sides, between the two malleoli and both the talus and calcaneus, which keep the joint surfaces in contact. The ankle joint, being cylindrical, has only one significant type of motion – dorsiflexion and plantarflexion – corresponding to flexion and extension in other joints.

The *subtalar* or talocalcaneal joint lies between the talus above and the calcaneus below. It has three articular surfaces: two anterior and medial and one posterior and lateral. Large numbers of ligaments join the two bones to each other and to all the adjacent bones. The axis of the joint is oblique, running primarily forwards but also upwards and medially. From a functional point of view, the importance of the subtalar joint is that it permits abduction and adduction (valgus/varus motion) of the hindfoot. When performing gait analysis, it is usually impossible to distinguish between movement at the ankle joint and that taking place at the subtalar joint and it is reasonable to refer to motion taking place at the 'ankle/subtalar complex'. This motion in normal individuals includes dorsiflexion, plantarflexion, hindfoot abduction and hindfoot adduction, plus a small amount of rotation about the long axis of the leg.

The *mid tarsal* joints lie between each of the tarsal bones and its immediate neighbors, making for a very complicated structure. The movement of most of these joints is very small, as there are ligaments crossing the joints and the joint surfaces are not shaped for large movements. As a result, the mid tarsal joints may be considered together to provide a flexible linkage between the hindfoot and the forefoot, which permits a small amount of movement in all directions.

The *tarsometatarsal* joints, between the cuboid and the cuneiforms proximally and the five metatarsals distally, are capable of only small gliding movements, because of the relatively flat joint surfaces and the ligaments binding the metatarsals to each other and to the tarsal bones. There are also joint surfaces between adjacent metatarsals, except for the medial one.

The *metatarsophalangeal* and *interphalangeal* joints consist of a convex proximal surface fitting into a shallow concave distal surface. The metatarsophalangeal joints permit abduction and adduction as well as flexion and extension; the interphalangeal joints are restricted by their ligaments to flexion and extension, the range of flexion being greater than that of extension. In walking, the most important movement in this region is extension at the metatarsophalangeal joints.

No description of the anatomy of the foot is complete without a mention of the arches. The bones of the foot are bound together by ligamentous structures, reinforced by muscle tendons, to make a flexible structure which acts like two strong curved springs, side by side. These are the longitudinal arches of the foot and they cause the body weight to be transmitted to the ground primarily through the calcaneus posteriorly and the metatarsal heads anteriorly. The midfoot transmits relatively little weight directly to the ground because it is lifted up, particularly on the medial side. The posterior end of both arches is the calcaneus. The *medial arch* (Fig. 1.6) goes upwards through the talus and then forward and gradually down again through the navicular and cuneiforms to the medial three metatarsals, which form the distal end of the arch. The *lateral arch* (Fig. 1.8) passes forwards from the calcaneus through the cuboid to the lateral two metatarsals.

Muscles and tendons

Muscles are responsible for movements at joints. Most muscles are attached to different bones at their two ends and cross over either one joint (*monarticular* muscle), two joints (*biarticular* muscle) or several joints (*polyarticular* muscle). In many cases the attachment to one of the bones covers a broad area, whereas at the other end it narrows into a *tendon*, which is attached to the

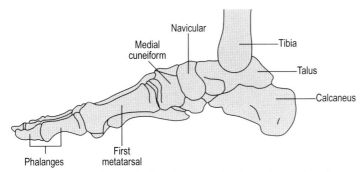

Fig. 1.6 Medial side of the right foot. The medial arch consists of the calcaneus, talus, navicular, cuneiforms and medial three metatarsals.

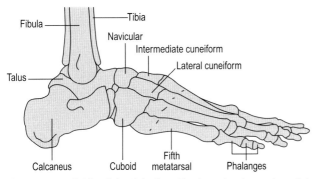

Fig. 1.7 Lateral side of the right foot. The lateral arch consists of the calcaneus, cuboid and lateral two metatarsals.

other bone. It is usual to talk about a muscle as having an 'origin' and an 'insertion', although these terms are not always clearly defined. Ligaments and tendons are obviously similar and frequently confused. As a general rule, ligaments connect two bones together, whereas tendons connect muscles to bones.

The account which follows gives very brief details of the muscles of the pelvis and lower limb, including their major actions. Most muscles also have secondary actions, which may vary according to the position of the joints, particularly with biarticular muscles. The larger and more superficial muscles are illustrated in Fig. 1.8.

Muscles acting only at the hip joint

1. *Psoas major* originates from the front of the lumbar vertebrae. *Iliacus* originates on the inside of the pelvis. The two tendons combine to form the *iliopsoas*, inserted at the lesser trochanter of the femur; the main action of these two muscles is to flex the hip.
2. *Gluteus maximus* originates from the back of the pelvis and is inserted into the back of the shaft of the femur near its top; it extends the hip.
3. *Gluteus medius* and *gluteus minimus* originate from the side of the pelvis and are inserted into the greater trochanter of the femur; they primarily abduct the hip.
4. *Adductor magnus, adductor brevis* and *adductor longus* all originate from the ischium and pubis of the pelvis. They insert in a line down the medial side of the femur and adduct the hip.
5. *Quadratus femoris, piriformis, obturator internus, obturator externus, gemellus superior* and *gemellus inferior* originate in the pelvis and insert close to the top of the femur; they all externally rotate the femur, although most also have secondary actions.
6. *Pectineus* originates on the pubis of the pelvis; it runs laterally and inserts on the front of the femur, near the lesser trochanter; it flexes and adducts the hip.

Internal rotation of the femur was not mentioned in the above list; it is achieved as a secondary action by gluteus medius, gluteus minimus, psoas major, iliacus, pectineus and tensor fascia lata (described below).

Muscles acting across the hip and knee joints

1. *Rectus femoris* originates from around the anterior inferior iliac spine of the pelvis and inserts into the quadriceps tendon; it flexes the hip, as well as being part of the *quadriceps*, a group of four muscles which extend the knee.
2. *Tensor fascia lata* originates from the pelvis close to the anterior superior iliac spine and is inserted into the iliotibial tract, a broad band of fibrous

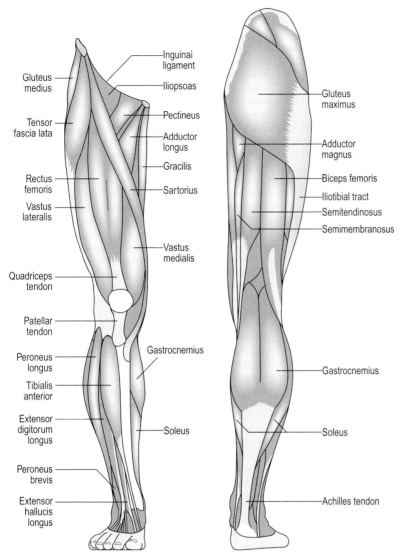

Fig. 1.8 Superficial muscles of the right leg.

tissue which runs down the outside of the thigh and attaches to the head of the fibula. The muscle abducts the hip and the knee.

3. *Sartorius* is a strap-like muscle originating at the anterior superior iliac spine of the pelvis and winding around the front of the thigh, to insert on the front of the tibia on its medial side; it is mainly a hip flexor.

4. *Semimembranosus* and *semitendinosus* are two of the *hamstrings*; both originate at the ischial tuberosity of the pelvis and are inserted into the medial condyle of the tibia; they extend the hip and flex the knee.

5. *Biceps femoris* is the third hamstring; it has two origins – the 'long head' comes from the ischial tuberosity and the 'short head' from the middle of

the shaft of the femur. It inserts into the lateral condyle of the tibia and is a hip extensor and knee flexor.

6. *Gracilis* runs down the medial side of the thigh from the pubis to the back of the tibia on its medial side; it adducts the hip and flexes the knee.

Muscles acting only at the knee joint

1. *Vastus medialis, vastus intermedius* and *vastus lateralis* are three elements of the quadriceps muscle. They all originate from the upper part of the femur, on the medial, anterior and lateral sides respectively. The fourth element of the quadriceps is rectus femoris, described above. The four muscles combine to become the quadriceps tendon. This surrounds the patella and continues beyond it as the patellar tendon, which inserts into the tibial tubercle. Quadriceps is the only muscle which extends the knee.
2. *Popliteus* is a small muscle behind the knee; it flexes and helps to unlock the knee by internally rotating the tibia at the beginning of flexion.

Muscles acting across the knee and ankle joints

1. *Gastrocnemius* originates from the back of the medial and lateral condyles of the femur; its tendon joins with that of the soleus (and sometimes also the plantaris) to form the *Achilles tendon*, which inserts into the back of the calcaneus. The main action of these muscles is to plantarflex the ankle, although the gastrocnemius is also a flexor of the knee.
2. *Plantaris* is a very slender muscle running deep to the gastrocnemius from the lateral condyle of the femur to the calcaneus; it is a feeble plantarflexor of the ankle.

Muscles acting across the ankle and subtalar joints

1. *Soleus* arises from the posterior surface of the tibia, fibula and the deep calf muscles. Its tendon joins with that of the gastrocnemius (and sometimes plantaris) to plantarflex the ankle. The soleus and gastrocnemius together are called the *triceps surae*.
2. *Extensor hallucis longus, extensor digitorum longus, tibialis anterior* and *peroneus tertius* form the anterior tibial group. They originate from the anterior aspect of the tibia and fibula and the interosseous membrane. The former two are inserted into the toes, which they extend; the latter two are inserted into the tarsal bones and raise the midfoot on the medial side (tibialis anterior) or lateral side (peroneus tertius). Tibialis anterior is the main ankle dorsiflexor; the others are weak dorsiflexors.
3. *Flexor hallucis longus, flexor digitorum longus, tibialis posterior, peroneus longus* and *peroneus brevis* are the deep calf muscles and all arise from the back of the tibia, fibula and interosseous membrane. The former two are flexors of the toes; the peronei are on the lateral side and evert the foot;

tibialis posterior is on the medial side and inverts it. All five muscles are weak ankle plantarflexors.

Muscles within the foot

1. *Extensor digitorum brevis* and the *dorsal interossei* are on the dorsum of the foot; the former muscle extends the toes and the latter muscles abduct and flex the toes.
2. *Flexor digitorum brevis, abductor hallucis* and *abductor digiti minimi* form the superficial layer of the sole of the foot; they flex the toes and abduct the big toe and the little toe, respectively.
3. *Flexor accessorius, flexor hallucis brevis* and *flexor digiti minimi brevis* form an intermediate layer in the sole of the foot; between them they flex all the toes.
4. The *adductor hallucis* is in two parts – the oblique and transverse heads. It adducts the big toe.
5. The *plantar interossei* and the *lumbricals* lie in the deepest layer of the sole of the foot; the former adduct and flex the toes, the latter flex the proximal phalanges and extend the distal ones.

The above five groups of muscles are known together as the *intrinsic muscles* of the foot.

Spinal cord and spinal nerves

The *spinal cord* is an extension of the brain and plays an active role in the processing of nerve signals. Like the brain itself, it consists of white matter, which is bundles of nerve fibers, and gray matter, which contains many cell bodies and nerve endings, where the synapses (connections) between nerve cells take place. The spinal cord lies within the spinal canal, which is formed in front by the vertebral bodies and behind by the neural arches of the vertebrae (Fig. 1.9). The vertebrae are divided into four groups: cervical (7 vertebrae), thoracic (12), lumbar (5) and sacral (5). It is usual to use abbreviated names; for example, the fourth thoracic vertebra is known as 'T4'.

The spinal cord is shorter than the spinal canal, terminating in adults at approximately the level of the first lumbar vertebra (L1) and in children a little lower. Beyond the end of the spinal cord is a bundle of nerves known as the *cauda equina*, which consists of those nerve roots which enter and leave the lower levels of the spinal canal (Fig. 1.10). There are eight cervical nerve roots but only seven cervical vertebrae; each nerve root except the eighth emerges above the correspondingly numbered vertebra. In the remainder of the spine, the nerve roots emerge below the correspondingly numbered vertebrae.

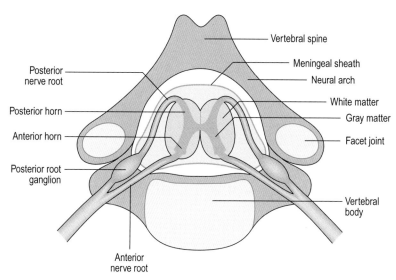

Fig. 1.9 Cross-section of vertebra, spinal cord and nerve roots.

The organization of the *neurons* (nerve cells) of the spinal cord and the peripheral nerves is extremely complicated. It is possible to give here only a brief outline, although further details will be given in the physiology section later in this chapter. The main neurons responsible for muscle contraction pass down from the brain as *upper motor neurons* in the 'descending' tracts of the spinal cord. At the appropriate spinal level, they enter the gray matter and connect with the *lower motor neurons*, also called *efferent* neurons. The axons (nerve fibers) of these cells pass out of the spinal cord through the *anterior root*, combine with other spinal roots and then split into smaller and smaller nerves, finally reaching the muscle itself.

Nerve fibers also pass in the opposite direction, from the muscles, skin and other structures to the spinal cord. They enter the spinal cord at the *posterior root*, having passed through the *posterior root ganglion*, a swelling which contains the cell bodies of the neurons. These *afferent* neurons transmit many different types of sensory information. Some connect with the nerve fibers which pass up the spinal cord to the brain in the 'ascending' tracts, while others synapse with other nerve cells at the same or nearby spinal levels. Connections within the spinal cord are responsible for the spinal reflexes, which will be referred to later.

When the spinal cord is damaged by accident or disease, the results depend both on the spinal level at which the damage occurred and on whether the cord was totally or partially transected (cut through). A wide variety of disabilities may result from incomplete destruction of the spinal cord. If the cord is totally transected, the upper motor neurons are unable to control the muscle groups at or below that level, so voluntary control of those muscles is lost. There is also a total loss of sensation below the level of the damage. However, at levels below the damaged area, there is usually preservation of

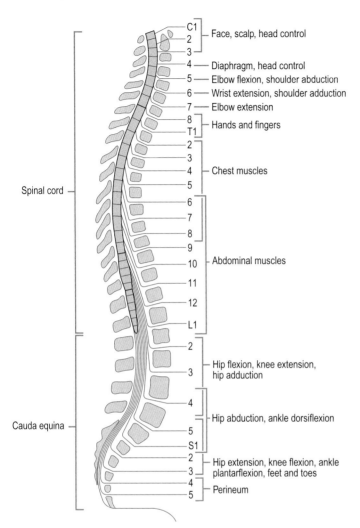

Fig. 1.10 Spinal cord and spinal nerves, with main functions served.

the lower motor neurons, the sensory nerves and the spinal reflexes. Injury to the vertebral column below L1 will damage the cauda equina, rather than the spinal cord. The cauda equina consists of lower motor neurons and sensory fibers and damage to it produces a totally different clinical picture from damage to the spinal cord itself.

Patients paralyzed at the level of the cervical spine are *tetraplegic* or *quadriplegic*, with paralysis of the arms and legs. With a cervical lesion above C4, the diaphragm is also paralyzed, making breathing difficult or impossible, and the chances of survival are poor. At the lower cervical levels, some arm or hand function is preserved. Where the spinal cord damage is at thoracic or lumbar level, only the legs are paralyzed and the patient is *paraplegic*. Where only the cauda equina is damaged, the patient has an incomplete paraplegia and may be able to walk wearing some form of orthosis (an external support, also known as a brace or caliper). The word 'orthotic' was once synonymous with 'orthosis' but current usage restricts it to orthotic insoles, used within the shoes. Patients with paralysis restricted to one side of the body are *hemiplegic*. Sometimes the suffix '-paretic' may be used in place of '-plegic'; it implies an incomplete paralysis.

The area of skin served by the sensory nerves from a particular spinal root is known as a *dermatome*. The distribution of the dermatomes for all the spinal nerves is shown in Fig. 1.11. In the legs, the anterior surface is innervated by the higher spinal segments and the posterior by the lower ones; loss of sensation from the buttocks and perineum is likely to follow spinal injury at almost any level.

Peripheral nerves

On emerging from the spinal cord, the spinal roots from adjacent levels form a network known as a *plexus*. The peripheral nerves which emerge from such a plexus usually contain nerve fibers from several adjacent spinal roots. The

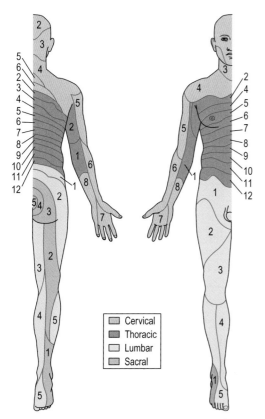

Fig. 1.11 Sensory distribution (dermatomes) of spinal nerve roots.

peripheral nerves supplying the muscles of walking all arise from either the *lumbar plexus* or the *sacral plexus*. Table 1.1 gives brief details of the motor and sensory distribution of the nerves arising from the lumbar plexus and Table 1.2 the corresponding information for the sacral plexus (sometimes called the lumbosacral plexus).

PHYSIOLOGY

Again, the text which follows is only intended to give an overview of the most important aspects of physiology which apply to gait. There are many good textbooks on the subject; the author uses one by Guyton (1991).

Table 1.1 Distribution of nerves arising from the lumbar plexus

Nerve	Origin	Motor	Sensory
Anterior lumbar nerves	L2–3	Psoas major	–
Iliohypogastric	T12–L1	Abdominal wall	Abdominal wall Lateral buttocks
Ilioinguinal	T12–L1	Abdominal wall	Abdominal wall Upper thigh Genitalia
Genitofemoral	L1–2	Genitalia	Upper thigh (anterior) Genitalia
Lateral femoral cutaneous	L2–3	–	Upper thigh (lateral)
Femoral	L2–4	Iliacus Pectineus Sartorius Rectus femoris Vastus lateralis Vastus intermedius Vastus medialis	Anterior thigh Medial thigh Medial leg Medial foot Hip joint Knee joint
–Saphenous	L2–4	–	Medial leg Medial foot Knee joint
Obturator	L2–4	Obturator externus Pectineus Adductor longus Adductor brevis Adductor magnus Gracilis	Medial thigh Hip joint Knee joint

Table 1.2 Distribution of nerves arising from the sacral plexus

Nerve	Origin	Motor	Sensory
Superior gluteal	L4–S1	Gluteus medius Gluteus medius Tensor fascia lata	–
Inferior gluteal	L5–S2	Gluteus maximus	–
Nerve to piriformis	S1–2	Piriformis	–
Nerve to quadratus femoris	L4–S1	Quadratus femoris Inferior gemellus	Hip joint
Nerve to obturator internus	L5–S2	Obturator internus Superior gemellus	–
Perforating cutaneous	S2–3	–	Medial buttock
Posterior cutaneous	S1–3	–	Inferior buttock Posterior thigh Upper calf
Sciatic	L4–S3	Biceps femoris Semimembranosus Semitendinosus Adductor magnus	Knee joint
–Tibial	L4–S3	Gastrocnemius Plantaris Soleus Popliteus Tibialis posterior Flex dig longus Flex hall longus	Lower leg (posterior) Posterior foot Lateral foot Knee joint Ankle joint
– –Medial plantar		Abductor hallucis Flex dig brevis Flex hall brevis	Medial foot Distal toes Tarsal joints
– –Lateral plantar		Remaining muscles of foot	Lateral foot Tarsal joints
– –Common peroneal	L4–S2	–	Knee joint
– –Superficial peroneal		Peroneus longus Peroneus brevis	Anterior leg Dorsal foot
– –Deep peroneal		Tibialis anterior Ext hall longus Ext dig brevis Ext dig longus Peroneus tertius	Great toe Second toe Ankle joint Tarsal joints
Pudendal	S2–4	Perineum	Genitalia

Nerves

Mention has already been made of the nerve cell or *neuron*, the basic element of the nervous system. Although neurons in different parts of the nervous system vary considerably in structure, they all consist of four basic elements (Fig. 1.12): *dendrites, cell body, axon* and *presynaptic endings*. Nerve impulses are

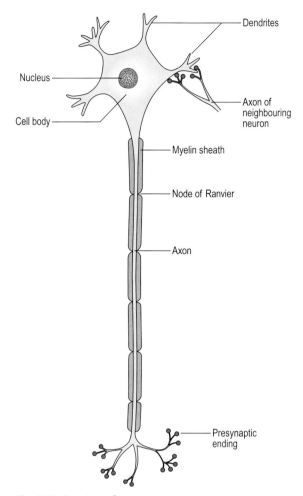

Nucleus

Cell body

Dendrites

Axon of neighbouring neuron

Myelin sheath

Node of Ranvier

Axon

Presynaptic ending

Fig. 1.12 Structure of a neuron.

conducted from the dendrites to the cell body and thence down the axon to the presynaptic endings. These contain very small packages of a chemical known as a *neurotransmitter*, which is released and crosses a small space known as a *synapse*, to stimulate the dendrite of another neuron. Within the brain and spinal cord, dendrites are stimulated to produce nerve impulses by the axons of other cells and in turn the nerve impulse sent along the axon stimulates the dendrites of other neurons. The peripheral nerves contain *motor neurons*, whose axons stimulate muscle fibers, and *sensory neurons*, in which the dendrites are stimulated by the sense organs.

The brain and spinal cord consist of millions of neurons, connected together in a vast and complex network. A single peripheral nerve consists of the axons and dendrites of hundreds or even thousands of individual neurons. The tissues of the brain, spinal cord and peripheral nerves also contain a number of other types of cell known as *neuroglia*, whose functions are either to provide physical support for the neurons or to perform a variety of maintenance functions.

The *upper motor neurons* arise in several different areas of the brain, but most notably in an area known as the motor cortex, and pass down the spinal cord to the appropriate level, crossing over to the other side at some point in their journey. Within the anterior horn of gray matter, the upper motor neurons synapse with the lower motor neurons, as well as with a large number of other neurons, which take part in the complex system of motor control.

The *lower motor neurons* or efferent neurons arise in the anterior horns of the spinal cord, emerge from the anterior spinal roots and pass down the peripheral nerves to the muscles. The axon usually branches at its distal end, where it synapses with the muscle cells at a number of *motor endplates*. The nerve impulse causes contraction of the muscle, by a process which will be described later.

The *sensory nerves* arise in the sense organs of the skin, joints, muscles and other structures. The sense organ itself stimulates the end of the dendrite of the afferent neuron. The dendrite usually commences as a number of branches; these come together and run up the peripheral nerve to enter the posterior root of the spinal cord. The cell body is in the *posterior root ganglion* (Fig. 1.9) and the axon runs from this ganglion into the spinal cord itself, usually terminating in the posterior horn of gray matter, where it synapses with other neurons. As well as the familiar sensations of touch, temperature, pain and vibration, sensory nerves also carry *proprioception* signals, which are used for feedback in the control of the limbs. These signals include the positions of the joints and the tension in the muscles and ligaments.

The term *nerve impulse* has been used above without explanation and it is now time to rectify this deficiency. The nature of the nerve impulse is a little difficult to grasp, since it is a complicated electrochemical process.

There are different concentrations of ions between the inside of cells (of all types) and the surrounding extracellular fluid. (Ions are atoms or molecules that have gained or lost one or more electrons, making them electrically charged.) The outside layer of a cell is known as the *cell membrane*; it is largely impermeable to sodium ions and any that leak in are 'pumped' out again. The inside of the cell contains large negatively charged ions, such as proteins, which are unable to pass through the cell membrane. The high concentration of positively charged sodium ions outside the cell, and of negative ions inside it, causes an automatic compensation, which results in a high concentration of potassium ions on the inside of the cell and of chloride ions outside. The inside of the cell thus has higher concentrations of potassium and large negative ions, while the outside has more sodium and chloride. The result of these imbalances in ionic concentration is a voltage difference between the inside and outside of the cell, across the thickness of the cell membrane. This *membrane potential* can be measured if a suitably small electrode is inserted.

The normal resting membrane potential for a neuron is around −70 mV, the negative sign indicating that the inside of the cell is negative with respect to the outside.

All body cells exhibit a membrane potential but nerve and muscle cells differ from other cells in that they can manipulate it, by altering the permeability of the cell membrane to sodium and potassium ions. This is the mechanism by which both nerve impulses and muscular contraction are propagated. If the membrane potential is lowered by about 20 mV, the membrane suddenly becomes extremely permeable to sodium ions, which enter rapidly from the extracellular fluid. While these ions are entering, the membrane potential is reversed to about +40 mV and it is said to be *depolarized*. The increase in permeability to sodium ions is shortlived and is followed by an increased permeability to potassium ions, which leave the cell, thus restoring the ionic balance and returning the membrane potential to −70 mV. The actual number of ions crossing the cell membrane is small and the overall composition of the cell is not affected to any appreciable extent; it is only when the sodium ions have entered, but before the potassium ions have left, that the membrane potential is reversed. This change in membrane potential by around 110 mV, from −70 mV to +40 mV, is known as an *action potential*.

Under normal circumstances, an action potential in a neuron begins in the synapses, in response to the neurotransmitters released from the presynaptic endings of the axons of other neurons. Some of these are excitatory, which means that they reduce the membrane potential, and some are inhibitory, in that they increase it. This combination of excitatory and inhibitory influences permits the addition and subtraction of nerve impulses. If the net effect of the various excitatory and inhibitory influences causes the membrane potential to fall by around 20 mV, an action potential will occur in that region of the neuron. This action potential spreads from its origin, crossing the cell body and running down the axon to its termination.

The action potential is an 'all-or-none' phenomenon, its size and shape being independent of the intensity of the stimulus, providing it is above the threshold; there are no 'larger' or 'smaller' action potentials. However, the spacing of the action potentials may vary; a nerve can pass action potentials one after another, in quick succession, or only occasionally and separated by long intervals. Thus it is the frequency of the nerve impulses, not their size, which carries the information on how hard the muscle is to be contracted, for example, or on the temperature of the skin.

Figure 1.13 shows an action potential passing along an axon from left to right. At its leading edge, sodium ions enter the axon, producing a region with reversed polarity. At the trailing edge of the action potential, potassium ions leave the axon and the membrane potential is restored. The depolarized region has a membrane potential of +40 mV, whereas the surrounding regions have a membrane potential of around −70 mV. This is equivalent to a tiny battery

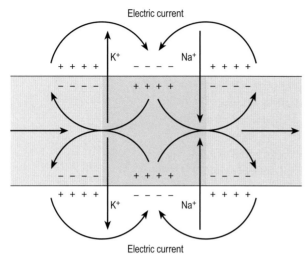

Fig. 1.13 Propagation of an action potential along an axon. Electric current flows from positive regions (+) to negative regions (–). The depolarized region is colored blue.

producing 110 mV and an electric current flows between the depolarized region and the surrounding normal regions of cell membrane. The passage of this electric current causes a drop in the membrane potential sufficient to generate an action potential in the normally polarized region in front, enabling the action potential to spread along the nerve. The region immediately behind an action potential becomes *refractory*, meaning that it cannot be stimulated again for a few milliseconds, so the action potential only moves in one direction.

The description so far has ignored the fact that many nerve fibers, particularly those required to send impulses quickly over long distances, are enclosed in a *myelin sheath*, as shown in Fig. 1.12. Myelin is a fatty substance which surrounds nerve fibers, both axons and dendrites, as a series of sleeves, with gaps between them known as *nodes of Ranvier*. Since myelin is an insulator, it prevents the electric current from passing through the cell membrane close to an area of depolarization, forcing it instead to pass through the next node of Ranvier, some distance along the nerve fiber. The effect of this is to cause the action potential to pass down the fiber in a series of jumps, known as *saltatory conduction*, which is much faster than the continuous propagation seen in unmyelinated fibers. A number of neurological diseases, most notably multiple sclerosis, are associated with loss of myelin from nerve fibers, with serious consequences to the functioning of the nervous system.

The speed at which nerve impulses travel depends on two things: the diameter of the nerve fiber and whether or not it is myelinated. Three speeds of fiber are found within the nervous system, known as types A, B and C. Type A fibers are all myelinated and are further divided by their conduction velocities into three:

- alpha (α), about 100 m/s
- beta (β), about 60 m/s
- gamma (γ), about 40 m/s.

Type B and C fibers are unmyelinated with conduction velocities around 10 m/s and 2 m/s respectively. The type A fibers are the most important in gait analysis, especially the alpha fibers which are used for the motor nerves to muscles and the faster sensory nerves such as touch. The gamma fiber is of particular importance in muscle physiology and will be referred to again later.

When an unmyelinated nerve fiber becomes damaged, recovery of function is usually impossible, because of the formation of scar tissue. For this reason, very little recovery of neuronal function takes place following damage to the brain or spinal cord, although function may be partially restored by the use of alternative neurological pathways. Myelinated fibers can recover, providing the cell body remains alive and the myelin sheaths remain in line; the nerve fiber regrows down the sheath at the rate of a few millimeters a week. In practice, if a complete nerve is divided and reconnected, most of the nerve fibers will enter the wrong myelin sheaths, although a sufficient number may be correctly connected to provide useful sensory and motor function.

Muscles

The human body contains three types of muscle: smooth, cardiac and skeletal. The description which follows is of *skeletal muscle*, also known as voluntary or striated muscle, which is responsible for the movement of the limbs.

A muscle is made up of hundreds of *fascicles* (Fig. 1.14), which in turn consist of hundreds of *muscle fibers*. These large multinucleated cells (cells with many nuclei) are the basic units of muscle tissue. The fiber is itself made up of hundreds of *myofibrils*, which have a characteristic striated (striped) appearance. The striations are due to a regular arrangement of *filaments*, which are made of two types of protein – *actin* and *myosin*. It is the sliding of these filaments past each other, by the formation and destruction of cross-bridges, which is responsible for muscle contraction.

The various light and dark bands in the myofibril are identified by letters. The thin, dark 'Z' line is the origin of the slender actin filaments (Fig. 1.15). These are interleaved with the thicker myosin filaments, which form the 'A' band. The 'I' band and 'H' zone change their width during muscular con-traction, as they represent the areas where the actin and myosin, respectively, are *not* overlapped – they were named before the process of contraction was understood!

There is an extremely complicated arrangement of membranes surrounding the myofibrils within the muscle fiber. It is responsible for the

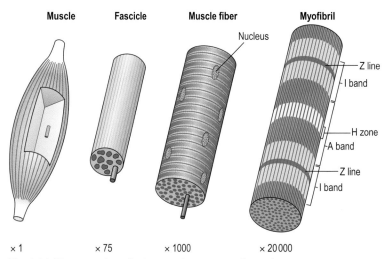

Muscle **Fascicle** **Muscle fiber** **Myofibril**

Nucleus

Z line
I band

H zone
A band
Z line
I band

× 1 × 75 × 1000 × 20 000

Fig. 1.14 Macroscopic and microscopic structure of muscle.

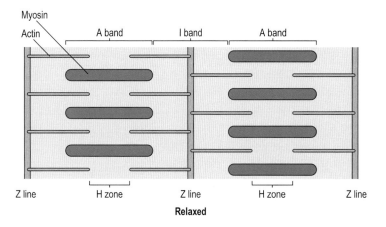

Myosin
Actin

A band | I band | A band

Z line | H zone | Z line | H zone | Z line

Relaxed

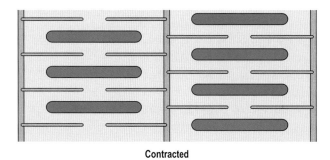

Contracted

Fig. 1.15 Sliding of actin and myosin filaments during muscular contraction.

transport of nutrients and waste products and the transmission of the muscle action potential. Outside the muscle fibers are the blood capillaries and the terminal branches of the motor nerves, which connect to the muscle fibers at *motor endplates*, also known as neuromuscular junctions. On average, a single motor nerve will connect to about 150 muscle fibers, the combination of the neuron and the muscle fibers it innervates being known as a *motor unit*.

When an action potential passes down a nerve to the motor endplate, it results in the release of the transmitter substance *acetylcholine* (ACH). This depolarizes the cell membrane of the muscle fiber and causes a spreading wave of depolarization. As this *muscle action potential* spreads throughout the muscle fiber, it causes the release of calcium ions, which are the trigger for muscle contraction. Cross-bridges form between the actin and myosin molecules, pulling them together. The tension is maintained for a brief period, then released if no further action potential occurs, the calcium ions being removed by the *calcium pump*. The electrical activity of muscle action potentials can be detected and is known as the *electromyogram* (EMG).

The energy for muscular contraction comes from the release of a high-energy phosphate group from a chemical known as *adenosine triphosphate* (ATP). The regeneration of ATP requires the expenditure of metabolic energy and a failure to keep up with the demand results in muscle fatigue. There are two metabolic pathways involved in regenerating ATP. One uses up chemicals stored within the cell (phosphocreatine and glucose), without the need for oxygen, and is known as *anaerobic*; the other requires oxygen and nutrients to enter the muscle fiber from the bloodstream and is known as *aerobic*. Anaerobic processes are quickly exhausted, although they can provide brief bursts of powerful contraction. For more sustained muscular effort, aerobic metabolism is required. Following anaerobic respiration, a muscle will have an *oxygen debt*, which will need to be 'repaid' by aerobic respiration, to remove lactic acid, which accumulates in the muscle.

If a single nerve impulse stimulates a muscle, it will respond, after a short pause known as the *latent period*, with a brief contraction known as a *twitch* (Fig. 1.16). If the motor nerve delivers a second nerve impulse during the latent period, it has no effect. If the nerve is repeatedly stimulated but there is sufficient time for one twitch to end before the next occurs, the force of contraction will increase over the first few twitches, a phenomenon known as *treppe*. If there is insufficient time for the muscle to relax before it is stimulated again, the force will build up as a *tetanus*. (The disease of the same name results in muscular contraction due to bacterial toxins.) The muscular contractions seen in gait are all tetanic. The force which a muscle is able to generate in a tetanic contraction depends on a number of factors, particularly the strength of stimulation, the cross-sectional area of the muscle, the speed of contraction and the direction of contraction. The greatest force is usually produced when the muscle length is close to its resting length. If a muscle shortens to its minimum length, its force of contraction falls to zero ('*active insufficiency*'). If the muscle becomes stretched well beyond its resting length,

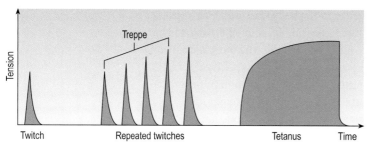

Fig. 1.16 Response of a single muscle fiber to single stimulation and to repeated stimulation at low and high frequencies.

it develops tension passively through stretching but little tension can be developed through active contraction ('*passive insufficiency*').

There are a number of different types of muscle fiber, the main subdivision being into types I and II. The type of muscle fiber depends on the type of stimulation reaching it down the motor nerve and because of this, all the fibers in a single motor unit are of the same type. *Type I fibers* (slow twitch) are dark in color, they contract and relax slowly and are fatigue resistant; they are used primarily for the sustained contractions used for posture control. *Type II fibers* (fast twitch) are pale in color, quick to contract and relax, and easily fatigued. They are mainly used for brief bursts of powerful contraction. Depending on their function in the body, different muscles have different proportions of fast and slow fibers. This is also seen in poultry, where the 'red meat' in the leg muscles is used for sustained contraction and the 'white meat' in the wing muscles for bursts of powerful contraction. A change in the stimulation pattern will cause a change in the fiber type in the course of a few weeks, despite the fact that the fiber types differ in the actual structure of the myosin. This ability to alter the fiber type becomes very important when electrical stimulation is used on paralyzed muscles.

When a muscle contracts, not all the motor units are active at the same time. If a stronger contraction is needed, further motor units are brought into use, a process known as *recruitment*.

If a muscle generates tension without changing its length, the contraction is known as *isometric*. If the muscle changes its length but the force of contraction remains the same, the contraction is *isotonic*. One normally thinks of a muscle shortening as it contracts – a *concentric contraction*. However, it is quite usual, particularly in gait, for a muscle to produce tension while it is lengthening – an *eccentric contraction*. For example, the quadriceps undergoes an eccentric contraction as you sit down. The muscle which is responsible for a particular action is known as an *agonist*. If two or more muscles act together, they are known as *synergists*; muscles which oppose agonists are known as *antagonists*. As a general rule, contraction of one set of muscles results in *reciprocal inhibition* of opposing muscles.

Muscle atrophy is the term used to describe the loss of bulk and strength of a muscle when it is not used. If the motor nerve is intact, the muscle fibers will become smaller but their numbers remain the same and subsequent restoration of muscle stimulation will lead to a full recovery of function. This happens, for example, when a limb is encased in plaster following a fracture. This type of muscle atrophy also occurs in spinal cord injury where the upper motor neurons are destroyed but the lower motor neurons remain intact. In contrast, if the lower motor neuron is destroyed, the muscle fibers shrink and become replaced by fibrous tissue. This leads to an irreversible form of muscle atrophy, such as is seen following poliomyelitis and after damage to the cauda equina or peripheral nerves.

Spinal reflexes

The lower motor neurons receive nerve impulses from both the brain and other neurons within the spinal cord. The two areas of the brain chiefly concerned with posture and movement are the *motor cortex*, which is responsible for voluntary movement, and the *cerebellum*, which is responsible for generating patterns of muscular activity. The motor cortex and its associated nerves are known as the *pyramidal system*; the cerebellum and some associated brain centers, with their associated nervous pathways, are known as the *extrapyramidal system*. Within the spinal cord itself, the influences of other neurons give rise to the *spinal reflexes*. There are also pattern generators for each limb within the spinal cord, which are capable of producing alternating flexion and extension.

The brain and higher centers exert an inhibitory influence on spinal reflexes, which as a result are often very weak in normal individuals. However, the reflexes may become very strong, due to the loss of this inhibition, in patients who have suffered damage to the brain or spinal cord.

One of the most important spinal reflexes is the *stretch reflex*, which is responsible for the knee-jerk, when the patellar tendon is struck by a small hammer. When a muscle is stretched, *stretch receptors* within it are stimulated, sending nerve impulses to the spinal cord along fast sensory neurons. Within the cord, these neurons synapse with and stimulate the lower motor neurons of the same muscle, causing it to contract. The stretch receptors are within the *muscle spindles* and attached to very small *intrafusal muscle fibers*, which are innervated by thin, relatively slow *gamma motor neurons*. These adjust the length of the spindle as the main muscle contracts and relaxes, so that it continues to work over the complete range of muscle lengths. The intrafusal fibers are also able to alter the 'sensitivity' of the stretch receptor. The stretch reflex provides a feedback system for maintaining the position of a muscle despite changes in the force applied to it.

The stretch reflex is unusual in that it involves only a single synapse, between the sensory and motor neurons, making it a *monosynaptic reflex*. Most reflexes are *polysynaptic*, involving many intermediate neurons and often involving neurons on both sides of the spinal cord and at more than one spinal level.

Partly because of the stretch reflex and partly through a continuous low level of activity in the motor neurons, most muscles show a certain amount of resistance to being stretched – this is known as *muscle tone*. In some individuals this effect is exaggerated, giving the clinical condition of *spasticity*, in which muscle tone is very high, small movements of the limb being opposed by strong muscular contractions. Spasticity is an important cause of gait abnormalities. It usually results from the loss of some or all of the inhibitory influence of the higher centers on the spinal reflexes and is often seen in patients with brain damage (as in cerebral palsy) or following damage to the spinal cord. A related phenomenon, also seen in gait, is *clonus* in which a muscle produces a series of contractions, one after the other, in response to being stretched.

Many different types of sensory organ in the tissues are responsible for spinal reflexes, those of particular importance in gait analysis being the muscle spindle, referred to above, and the *Golgi organ*. The latter is a stretch receptor in tendons which inhibits muscular contraction if the force applied to the tendon, either actively or passively, becomes dangerously large. Pain receptors in the limb may elicit the *flexor withdrawal reflex*, in which the flexor muscles contract and the extensors relax, hopefully to remove the limb from whatever is causing the pain. There is also a *crossed extensor reflex*, where contraction of flexors on one side is accompanied by contraction of extensors on the other. However, this is very weak in humans, even after spinal cord transection.

Motor control

Walking is accomplished through a complex and coordinated pattern of nerve signals, sent to the muscles, which in turn move the joints, the limbs and the remainder of the body. The 'central pattern generator', which produces this pattern of nerve impulses, is not located in a single place but consists of networks of neurons in various parts of the brain and spinal cord. Much of the research in this area has been done on experimental animals but there is some evidence that human locomotion is organized in a similar fashion to that in cats, where a rhythm-generating system within the spinal cord is controlled by neural input from 'higher levels' in the brain and receives feedback from sensors in the muscles, joints and skin of the legs (Duysens & Van de Crommert, 1998).

BIOMECHANICS

Biomechanics is a scientific discipline which studies biological systems, such as the human body, by the methods of mechanical engineering. Since gait is a mechanical process which is performed by a biological system, it is appropriate to study it in this way. Mechanical engineering is a vast subject but the descriptions which follow are limited to those aspects which are most relevant to gait analysis, especially time, mass, force, center of gravity, moments of force, and motion, both linear and angular. The science of biomechanics can be extremely mathematical but the basic principles are easy to grasp and the section ends with a worked example to illustrate this. A good text on the scientific basis of movement is Gowitzke & Milner (1988).

Time

The second (s) and the millisecond (ms) are the primary units for time measurement in biomechanics, although it is still fairly common to find walking speed quoted in meters per minute or even miles per hour. When repeated events occur at short intervals of time, it is usual to quote a 'frequency' in hertz (abbreviated 'Hz'), 1 Hz being one cycle per second. For example, a typical television-based gait analysis system might measure the positions of markers on a patient's limbs at 50 Hz (corresponding to an interval between samples of 20 ms) and to sample the ground reaction force and EMG at 500 Hz (2 ms interval between samples). The relationship between sample interval and frequency is given by:

Interval (ms) = 1000/frequency (Hz)

Mass

As we all live in the Earth's gravitational field, we normally use the terms mass and weight to mean the same thing. However, there is a clear distinction between them. The *mass* of an object is the amount of matter contained in it, which does not depend on whether any gravity is present, whereas *weight* is the force exerted by gravity on the object. For example, in an orbiting spacecraft there is no gravity and all objects are weightless, although they still have mass. This means that you are still likely to be injured if someone throws a moon-rock at you inside a spacecraft, even though it doesn't 'weigh' anything! We casually talk about measuring our body 'weight' in kilograms (kg) or pounds but this is incorrect in scientific terms, as these are units of mass, not of force.

Force

We are all familiar in general terms with the concept of force but the scientist uses the term in a particular way. Force is a *vector* quantity, which means that it has both magnitude and direction, in contrast to *scalar* quantities, such as temperature, which have only magnitude. The internationally agreed system for scientific measurement is the Système International (SI). The unit of force in this system is the *newton* (N). The force applied by normal earth gravity to a mass of 1 kg is 9.81 N; one newton is the force exerted by gravity on a mass of about 102 g or 3½ ounces. This is easily visualized as being the weight of an average size apple! The earlier imperial and metric units of force were confusing and are best avoided; conversions will be found in Appendix 2. The direction of a force vector may be stated in any convenient manner, for example 20 N downwards or 140 N at 30° to the x-axis. However, the direction should never be omitted, unless it is obvious.

The whole science of mechanical engineering is based on the three laws of force propounded by Sir Isaac Newton, which may be paraphrased as follows.

Newton's first law: A body will continue in a state of rest, or of uniform motion in a straight line, unless it is acted upon by an external force.

Newton's second law: An external force will cause a body to accelerate in the direction of the force. The acceleration (a) is equal to the size of the force (F) divided by the mass (m) of the object, as in the equation:

$a = F/m$

Newton's third law: To every action there is a reaction, which is equal in magnitude and opposite in direction.

Neglecting the strange behavior of atomic and subatomic particles, all physical systems simultaneously obey all three of Newton's laws.

It is easy to remember which law is which if you first imagine a brick, just floating in space (first law); then someone pushes it and it accelerates (second law); as it is accelerating, the brick pushes back on whoever or whatever is pushing it (third law).

It is easy to see that a single force acting in one direction can be balanced out by an equal force acting in the opposite direction. A much more common situation, however, is to have a number of forces acting in different directions which, taken together, balance each other out. Providing direction is taken into account, it is possible to add and subtract force vectors, as it is with any other vectors such as velocity or acceleration. To understand how this is possible, it is necessary to appreciate the fact that a single force, acting in a single direction, can be exactly equivalent to a number of different forces acting in other directions. Conversely, any number of separate forces can be represented by an appropriate single force.

The technique used to convert a single force into two forces, acting in different directions, is known as *resolving into components*. Fig. 1.17 shows how the force F can be represented by two smaller forces, F_x and F_y, acting at right angles to each other. The magnitude of these forces is given by the formulae:

$$F_x = F \times \cos a$$
$$F_y = F \times \sin a$$

where a is the angle between F and F_x.

The converse process, that of combining F_x and F_y to produce F, can be performed using these formulae:

Magnitude: $F = \sqrt{(F_x^2 + F_y^2)}$

Angle: $a = \tan^{-1}(F_y/F_x)$

In order to combine forces, they are first resolved into components, using a common system of directions. Next, all the x components are added together and so are all the y components. The resulting totals are then used to find the single equivalent force. This is illustrated in Fig. 1.18, where two forces, A and B, are combined to give a resultant force R. First, A and B are resolved into components (A_x, A_y, B_x and B_y). The algebraic sum of the x components gives the x component of the resultant and similarly with the y components. Since A_x and B_x are in opposite directions, their algebraic sum is actually their difference. The resultant, R, is then obtained by recombining the x and y components.

When resolving a force into components, it is not necessary for the two components to be at right angles, although it makes the calculations much easier, since a triangle containing a right angle lends itself to simple geometrical and trigonometrical methods.

Figure 1.19 shows how graphical methods can be used to combine two forces, A and B, to give a single resultant force, R. The two forces are drawn as

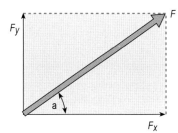

Fig. 1.17 Resolution of force F into two components at right angles: F_x and F_y.

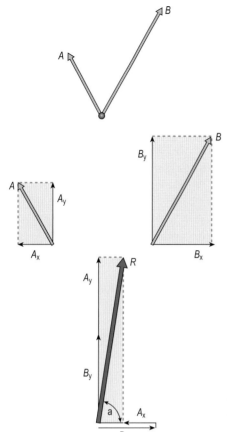

Fig. 1.18 Resolution of force *A* into A_x and A_y and force *B* into B_x and B_y. Algebraic addition of A_x and B_x horizontally, and of A_y and B_y vertically, gives the resultant, *R*.

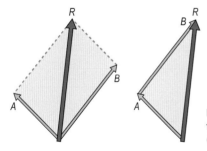

Fig. 1.19 Determination of resultant force, *R*, from forces *A* and *B* by parallelogram of forces (left) and triangle of forces (right).

a scale diagram, with the correct angle between them, the length of the line representing the magnitude of the force. On the left, *A* and *B* are used to draw a parallelogram, the diagonal of which shows the magnitude and direction of *R*; this is the *parallelogram of forces*. On the right, the *triangle of forces* is shown. This does not directly represent the physical arrangement of the forces, since if force *A* is drawn first, force *B* is drawn starting at its tip, not its base. The resultant force *R* is represented by the line which completes the triangle, by joining the base of A to the tip of B. Both the triangle of forces and the parallelogram of forces give the same result, as does the method illustrated in Fig. 1.18; it is a matter of convenience which one is used.

It follows from Newton's second law that if an object is not accelerating, there can be no net force acting on it. Any forces which are acting on the object must be balanced out by other, equal and opposite forces. If the forces do not appear to balance, yet the object is not accelerating or decelerating, there must be at least one force which has not been taken into account. This is illustrated in Fig. 1.20, which shows a complicated system of forces in use for the treatment of a fracture of the femur by the old-fashioned method of balanced traction. Such problems are conveniently approached by drawing a *free body diagram* where all the forces are drawn as acting on a shapeless 'lump', floating in space, and in which the sum of all the forces in any given direction must be zero. It can be seen that the forces from the traction system do not balance out; the missing force is the friction which prevents the patient from sliding down the bed. It can be found by a graphical method which is an extension of the triangle of forces or it can be calculated by resolving all the forces into vertical and horizontal components, calculating the 'missing'

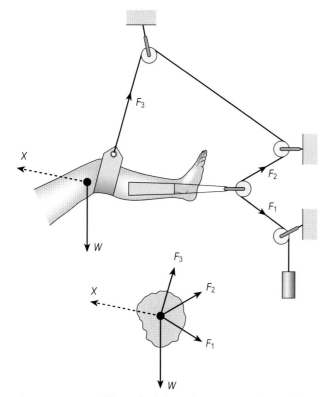

Fig. 1.20 System of forces for balanced traction. Neglecting friction in the pulleys, F_1, F_2 and F_3 all equal the traction weight. W is the weight of the leg and X the reaction force on the patient. The equivalent free body diagram is shown below.

element of each and then combining these components to give the magnitude and direction of the missing force.

Center of gravity

Although the mass of any object is distributed throughout every part of it, it is frequently convenient, as far as the effects of an applied force are concerned, to imagine that the whole mass is concentrated at a single point, which should be called the center of mass but is more usually called the *center of gravity* (C of G). For a regular shape, such as a cube, made of a uniform material, it is easy to see that the center of gravity must be at the geometric center. However, for irregular and changing shapes, such as the human body, it may be necessary to determine it by direct measurement. It is also possible to determine the center of gravity of every part of the body separately and to find the center of gravity of the whole body by adding these together (by a method which is beyond the scope of this book). It is frequently stated that the center of gravity of the body is just in front of the lumbosacral junction. This is approximately true for a person standing in the anatomical position but any movement of the body will move the center of gravity. It is not even necessary for the center of gravity to remain within the body; the center of gravity of someone bending down to touch their toes will usually be outside the body, in front of the top of the thigh (Fig. 1.21). An interesting example of this is the technique used by skilled high-jumpers, who curve the body in such a way that although each part of the body in turn passes *over* the bar, the center of gravity actually passes *under* it!

Moment of force

If an adult wishes to play with a small child on a seesaw, he will have to sit much closer to the pivot in order to balance the weight of the child (Fig. 1.22). The action which tends to unbalance the seesaw is the *moment of force*, which is calculated by multiplying the magnitude of the force by its perpendicular distance from the fulcrum or pivot point, this distance commonly being referred to as the *lever arm* or *moment arm*. The 'moment of force' may also be referred to as the 'torque', the 'turning moment' or simply the 'moment'. The formula for calculating the moment of force is:

$$M = F \times D$$

where M is the moment of force (in newton-meters, N·m), F is the force (in newtons, N) and D is the distance (in meters, m).

For the system to be in equilibrium (that is, for the seesaw to balance), *the sum of the clockwise moments of force must equal the sum of the anticlockwise*

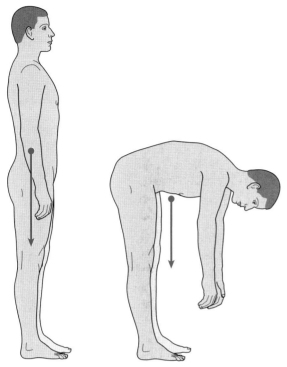

Fig. 1.21 Center of gravity when standing and when bending.

moments. In Fig. 1.22, if the child has a mass of 40 kg, she will exert a force due to gravity (F_c) of:

40 kg × 9.81 m/s^2 = 392.4 N

If her distance (D_c) from the fulcrum is 4 m, she exerts an anticlockwise moment of:

392.4 N × 4 m = 1569.6 N·m

A 70 kg adult will produce a downward force (F_a) of:

70 kg × 9.81 m/s^2 = 686.7 N

This will produce an opposing clockwise moment of 1569.6 N·m if he sits at a distance (D_a) from the fulcrum of:

1569.6 N·m/686.7 N = 2.29 m

The definition of a moment of force refers to the perpendicular distance from the fulcrum. This is very important if opposing moments are produced by

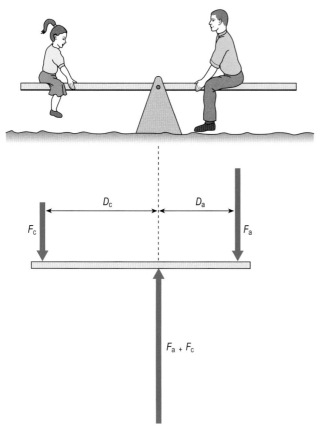

Fig. 1.22 The adult on the seesaw will balance the child if the force F_a multiplied by the distance D_a equals the force F_c multiplied by the distance D_c.

forces which act in different directions. Figure 1.23 illustrates the moments of force about the knee joint when standing with the knee bent. F_1, the weight of the body above this point, is acting at a perpendicular distance 'a' from the point of loadbearing. The quadriceps tendon is pulling at an oblique angle relative to the vertical and the moment of force it provides is the product of the tension in the tendon, F_2, and the perpendicular distance 'b'. It will be noted that the presence of the patella increases the value of b and hence reduces the muscle force needed to produce a given moment of force. For equilibrium, the two moments $(F_1 \times a)$ and $(F_2 \times b)$ must be equal.

The measurement and interpretation of moments of force are essential for the full understanding of normal and pathological gait. 'Active' internal moments are generated by muscular contraction (concentric, isometric or eccentric). 'Passive' internal moments are generated by bone-on-bone forces and by tension in the soft tissues, especially ligaments. Moments may also be transmitted from adjacent joints. External moments (sometimes referred to as 'reaction moments') are generally due to gravitational forces. Modern gait analysis systems are able to measure the 'net moment' at the major joints

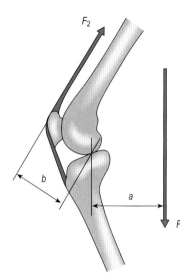

Fig. 1.23 The moment of force due to gravity, F_1 multiplied by a, is opposed by contraction of the quadriceps, producing a moment of force F_2 multiplied by b.

during walking, which is the sum of all the active and passive moments present. Unfortunately, this cannot generally be used to calculate the contraction force of a particular muscle, because there is frequently more than one muscle contracting. An example of this is 'co-contraction' at the hip joint, where flexor and extensor muscles contract at the same time, to increase the stability of the joint (Park *et al.*, 1999).

Unfortunately, some confusion exists in the literature, because a term like 'flexor moment' is often used without stipulating whether it refers to an internal or external moment. Contraction of a flexor muscle generates an *internal* flexor moment. In contrast, an *external* flexor moment attempts to flex the joint and is likely to be resisted by the contraction of extensor muscles. To avoid such confusion, it is essential to make it clear whether any moment is internal or external. The gait analysis community now tends to use internal moments, a convention which has been adopted in this book, although the important textbook by Perry (1992) used external moments.

A *couple* is a moment which is produced by two equal forces which are parallel to each other but acting in opposite directions. The forces cancel each other out as far as producing linear motion is concerned (displacement or acceleration) but work together to produce rotation about a point between them. An example of this is the 'plantarflexion/knee extension couple', referred to in Chapter 2 and Chapter 6, which is present in normal walking and exists in an exaggerated form in some pathological gaits.

In the same way that Newton's third law states that every force is opposed by another 'equal and opposite' force, every moment of force is opposed by an equal and opposite moment. It is impossible to generate a moment unless there is something to 'push back' with an opposing moment. The consequence of this for gait analysis is that if an external force generates a moment at a particular joint (attempting to flex the knee, for example), there *must* be a corresponding internal moment, generated within the joint, to oppose it. In the case of the knee, only the quadriceps muscles can provide an internal extensor moment, although for most joints both muscles and stretched ligaments can generate internal moments.

Any object which is supported by the ground will remain stable so long as the *line of gravity* (the line of force passing vertically downwards from the center of gravity) remains within the area on the ground which is supporting it. Should the line of gravity stray outside this area, one of two things can happen: it may automatically correct itself, as happens with a self-righting lifeboat, or it may fall over, as will happen with a pencil balanced on its point. The former is a *stable equilibrium*, where a degree of imbalance produces 'restoring' moments, which push the object back towards the balanced position. The latter is an *unstable equilibrium*, where the moments act to increase the imbalance. When walking at moderate speeds, a further condition exists – a *dynamic equilibrium*, where from instant to instant the equilibrium is unstable but before there has been time to fall, the area of support is moved and equilibrium is restored.

The measurement of the moments generated about the joints of the lower limbs is an important part of scientific gait analysis. Such moments may be expressed in their original units (e.g. newton-meters) or they may be 'normalized' by dividing by body mass, changing the units to newton-meters per kilogram, to make it easier to compare results between individuals of different sizes. Although there is no general agreement on the best method of accomplishing such normalization (Pierrynowski & Galea, 2001; Stansfield *et al.*, 2003), it seems reasonable to normalize forces with reference to body mass and moments with reference to both body mass and either height or limb length.

Linear motion

The *velocity* of a moving object is the rate at which its position changes, which usually means the distance it covers in a given time. This is, of course, similar to the everyday concept of speed, except that velocity is a vector and thus has direction as well as magnitude. In measuring gait, the usual unit for velocity is meters per second, which can be abbreviated to either m/s or $m \cdot s^{-1}$. Sometimes other units are used, such as meters per minute or kilometers per hour, but the SI units are to be preferred.

Acceleration is the rate at which velocity changes; the change may be in either magnitude or direction. An unchanging velocity has an acceleration of zero; a decrease in velocity may be known as negative acceleration, deceleration or retardation. If the velocity is measured in meters per second, the acceleration will be in meters per second per second, abbreviated to m/s^2 or $m \cdot s^{-2}$. The acceleration due to gravity has already been mentioned; it has a value of 9.81 m/s^2.

The relationships between velocity, acceleration and distance traveled are given by four equations:

$$v = u + at$$
$$s = \tfrac{1}{2}\,(ut + vt)$$
$$s = ut + \tfrac{1}{2}\,at^2$$
$$v^2 - u^2 = 2\,as$$

where u is the initial velocity (in meters per second, m/s)
v is the final velocity (in meters per second, m/s)
a is the acceleration (in meters per second per second, m/s^2)
t it the time (in seconds, s)
s is the distance traveled (in meters, m).

The worked example at the end of this chapter uses one of these equations.

Circular motion

An object which is rotating has an *angular velocity* and if the angular velocity changes, there is an *angular acceleration*, such as when a wheel, rotating on its axle, either speeds up or slows down. In walking, the leg has an angular velocity and undergoes angular acceleration and retardation. Every rotating object has an angular velocity, even if it is not attached to an axle or fulcrum, and a change in that angular velocity is an angular acceleration. In the same way that linear acceleration depends on the presence of a force, angular acceleration will only occur if there is an application of a moment of force.

The detailed mathematics of angular velocity and angular acceleration are beyond the scope of this book, but it is worth saying a few words about the general concepts. Angular velocity is measured by the angle turned per unit time, usually in degrees per second or radians per second. Angular acceleration is similarly expressed in degrees (or radians) per second per second. The radian is an obscure unit to non-mathematicians; it is the ratio, within the arc of a circle, of the length of the arc to the radius of the circle. There are 2π radians in a complete circle, giving the relationship:

$$1\ \text{rad} = 180°/\pi = 57.296°$$

When a force applied to an object produces an angular acceleration, the acceleration does not depend solely on the size of the force and the mass of the object, as it does with linear motion. It also depends on the way in which the mass is distributed about the center of gravity, a property known as the *moment of inertia*. An object with the mass concentrated around the outside, such as a flywheel, has a much higher moment of inertia than one with the mass concentrated around the center, such as a cannon ball. If a flywheel and a cannon ball have the same mass and are spinning with the same angular velocity, the flywheel will be much more difficult to stop rotating than the cannon ball, because of its higher moment of inertia.

Inertia and momentum

The term *inertia* is used to describe the resistance offered by a body to any attempt to set it in motion or to stop it if it is already moving. It is a descriptive term, rather than a measured physical quantity. In the case of linear motion, it results from the mass of the object; in the case of rotational motion, it results from the moment of inertia.

Momentum exists in two forms – linear and angular. The *linear momentum* (generally just called 'momentum') of a moving object is calculated by multiplying its velocity by its mass. A force applied to the object will cause it to change its velocity and hence its momentum. Another way of expressing Newton's second law is to say that the force is equal to the rate of change of momentum. The *angular momentum* of a rotating object is calculated by multiplying its angular velocity by its moment of inertia. A law of conservation of momentum exists, which states that momentum (both linear and angular) cannot be created or destroyed, merely transferred from one object to another.

Momentum has received little attention in gait analysis in the past but transfers of momentum are involved at a number of key events of the gait cycle, including the heelstrike transient and the end of the swing phase, both of which will be described in more detail in Chapter 2.

Kinetics and kinematics

The terms kinetics and kinematics are commonly used in gait analysis and they deserve some explanation. *Kinetics* is the study of forces, moments, masses and accelerations, but without any detailed knowledge of the position or orientation of the objects involved. For example, an instrument known as a force platform is used in gait analysis to measure the force beneath the foot during walking, but it gives no information on the position of the limb or the angle of the joints. *Kinematics* describes motion, but without reference to the forces involved. An example of a kinematic instrument is a camera, which can be used to observe the motion of the trunk and the limbs during walking, but which gives no information on the forces involved. It is obvious that for an adequate quantitative description of an activity such as walking, both kinetic and kinematic data are needed.

Work, energy and power

One of the remarkable features of normal gait is how energy is conserved by means of a number of optimizations. Abnormal gait patterns involve a loss of these optimizations, which may result in excessive energy expenditure and hence fatigue. The measurement, during walking, of energy transfers at individual joints and overall energy consumption is an important component of scientific gait analysis.

There is a subtle difference in viewpoint between the physical scientist and the biologist as far as work, energy and power are concerned. To the physical scientist, *work* is done when a force moves an object a certain distance. It is calculated as the product of the force and the distance; if a force of two newtons moves an object three meters, the work done is:

$$2\,N \times 3\,m = 6\,J\ (joules)$$

The *joule* could also be called a newton-meter, but this would cause confusion with the identically named unit which is used to measure moment of force. *Energy* is the capacity to do work and is also measured in joules. It exists in two basic forms: *potential* or stored energy and *kinetic* or movement energy. In walking, there are alternating transfers between potential and kinetic energy, which will be described in Chapter 2. *Power* is the rate at which work is done; a rate of one joule per second is a *watt*, which is familiar to users of electrical appliances.

The reason biologists regard these matters slightly differently from physical scientists is that muscles can use energy without shortening, in other words without doing any physical work. The potential energy stored in the muscles, in the form of ATP, is converted to mechanical energy in response to the muscle action potential. This energy is still used, even in an eccentric contraction, where the muscle actually gets longer while developing a force, which in physical terms is negative work. In other words, while everyone agrees that walking uphill involves the doing of work, the physicist might expect someone walking downhill to gain energy, whereas in reality the muscles are still activated and metabolic energy is still consumed. Even if a muscle shortens as it contracts, in a concentric contraction, the conversion of metabolic energy to mechanical energy is relatively inefficient, with a typical efficiency of around 25%. The old unit for measuring metabolic energy was the Calorie (the capital C indicating 1000 calories or 1 kilocalorie); the conversion factor is 4200 J or 4.2 kJ equals one Calorie (see Appendix 2).

The calculation of the mechanical power generated at joints has become an important part of the biomechanical study of gait. In a rotary movement, when a joint flexes or extends, the power is calculated as the product of the moment of force and the angular velocity, omega (ω):

$$P \text{ (watts)} = M \text{ (newton-meters)} \times \omega \text{ (radians per second)}$$

In Chapter 2, reference will be made to the power exchanges across the hip, knee and ankle joints at different stages of the gait cycle. When a muscle is contracting concentrically (e.g. a flexor muscle contracts while a joint is flexing), power is generated. If a muscle contracts eccentrically (e.g. a flexor muscle contracts while a joint is extending), it absorbs power. If a muscle contracts isometrically (e.g. a flexor muscle contracts while the joint angle is unchanging), no power exchange takes place. Although, in the gait cycle, power generation and absorption are often due to muscle contraction, it is important to realize that the stretching of ligaments and other soft tissues also involves power exchange. If a ligament is stretched, it absorbs power, with a resulting storage of potential energy. Some or all of this stored energy may be released later, with a resulting power generation.

In gait analysis, it is common practice to 'normalize' joint power by dividing it by body mass, giving a unit of watts per kilogram, in a similar way to the treatment of joint moments (mentioned above).

Worked example

As an example of the biomechanical principles outlined above, consider the mechanics involved when 'Wonder Woman' (one of the fictional 'superheroes') jumps from the ground to the top of a building 10 m (32 ft 10 in) high. In order to perform this superhuman feat, she must leave the ground with sufficient velocity to reach the top of the building, despite the deceleration produced by gravity. The distance to be traveled (s) is 10 m; the initial velocity (u) is unknown; the final velocity (v) is zero and the acceleration (a) is −9.81 m/s^2, which is the acceleration due to gravity, negative because it opposes the movement. The substitution of these values in the equation:

$$v^2 - u^2 = 2\,as$$

gives the initial velocity (u) as 14.0 m/s.

In order to achieve the necessary velocity, Wonder Woman must accelerate from being stationary in the crouched position to a velocity of 14.0 m/s in the fully stretched position, as her feet leave the ground. The center of gravity of the body, in making this jump, moves through a vertical distance (s) of 0.7 m. The initial velocity (u) is zero, the final velocity (v) is 14.0 m/s. Substituting these values in the equation used above gives the average acceleration (a) as being 140 m/s^2, or about 14 times the acceleration due to gravity, and the duration of the acceleration as 0.1 seconds.

To achieve this acceleration requires a force acting vertically upwards on the center of gravity. The force is given by the equation:

$$F = m \times a$$

which follows from Newton's second law, where the force (F) is equal to the body mass (m) multiplied by the acceleration (a). If her body mass is 50 kg, the force is: 50 kg × 140 m/s² = 7000 N or 7 kN.

Neglecting the small contribution made by swinging the arms, this force is applied to the center of gravity of the body by extension of the two knees. When the knee is flexed to a right angle, about halfway through the acceleration, the center of gravity is about 0.4 m behind the knee joint, whereas the quadriceps tendon is only 0.06 m in front of it. To apply an upward force of 7 kN to the center of gravity, the moment of force required to be generated by each knee is: 7 kN × 0.4 m/2 = 1.4 kN·m.

Since the sum of the clockwise and anticlockwise moments must be equal, each quadriceps must generate a force of: 1.4 kN·m/0.06 m = 23.3 kN, or about 48 times body weight. Needless to say, only someone like Wonder Woman can generate quite such large forces in the quadriceps tendon, mere mortals having to settle for about a fifth as much!

The knee extends from about 160° of flexion to 0° in 0.1 seconds; its angular velocity is thus 1600° per second, or close to 30 radians per second. The power generated is the product of the moment of force and the angular velocity, which for the moment calculated above is: 1.4 kN·m × 30 rad/s = 42 kW. This contrasts with a power generation at the joints in normal walking of 100–300 watts.

References and suggestions for further reading

Duysens J, Van de Crommert HWAA. (1998) Neural control of locomotion; part 1: the central pattern generator from cats to humans. *Gait and Posture* **7**: 131–141.

Gowitzke BA, Milner M. (1988) *Scientific Bases of Human Movement*, 3rd edn. Baltimore, MD: Williams & Wilkins.

Guyton AC. (1991) *Textbook of Medical Physiology*, 8th edn. Philadelphia, PA: W.B. Saunders.

Palastanga N, Field D, Soames R. (1989) *Anatomy and Human Movement*. Oxford: Heinemann.

Pollo FE, Jackson RW, Komdeur P et al. (2003) Measuring dynamic knee motion with an instrumented spatial linkage device. Gait and Clinical Movement Analysis Society, Eighth Annual Meeting, Wilmington, Delaware, USA, pp. 15–16.

Park S, Krebs DE, Mann W. (1999) Hip muscle co-contraction: evidence from concurrent in vivo pressure measurement and force estimation. *Gait and Posture* **10**: 211–222.

Perry J. (1992) *Gait Analysis: Normal And Pathological Function*. Thorofare, NJ: Slack Incorporated.

Pierrynowski MR, Galea V. (2001) Enhancing the ability of gait analyses to differentiate between groups: scaling gait data to body size. *Gait and Posture* **13**: 193–201.

Stansfield BW, Hillman SJ, Hazlewood ME et al. (2003) Normalization of gait data in children. *Gait and Posture* **17**: 81–87.

Normal gait

2

In order to understand pathological gait, it is necessary first to understand normal gait, since this provides the standard against which the gait of a patient can be judged. However, there are two pitfalls which need to be borne in mind when using this approach. Firstly, the term 'normal' covers both sexes, a wide range of ages and an even wider range of extremes of body geometry, so that an appropriate 'normal' standard needs to be chosen for the individual who is being studied. If results from an elderly female patient are compared with normal data obtained from physically fit young men, there will undoubtedly be large differences, whereas comparison with data from healthy elderly women may show the patient's gait to be well within normal limits which are appropriate to her sex and age. The second pitfall is that even though a patient's gait differs in some way from normal, it does not follow that this is in any way undesirable or that efforts should be made to turn it into a 'normal' gait. Many gait abnormalities are a compensation for some problem experienced by the patient and, although abnormal, they are nonetheless useful.

Having said all that, it is very important to understand normal gait and the terminology which is used to describe it, before going on to look at pathological gait. The chapter starts with a very brief historical review and then gives an overview of the gait cycle, before going on to study in detail how the different parts of the locomotor system are used in walking.

WALKING AND GAIT

As walking is such a familiar activity, it is difficult to define it without sounding pompous. However, it would be remiss not to attempt a definition.

Normal human walking and running can be defined as 'a method of locomotion involving the use of the two legs, alternately, to provide both support and propulsion'. In order to exclude running, we must add '... at least one foot being in contact with the ground at all times'. Unfortunately, this definition excludes some forms of pathological gait which are generally regarded as being forms of walking, such as the 'three-point step-through gait' (see Fig. 3.21), in which there is an alternate use of two crutches and either one or two legs. It is probably both unreasonable and pointless to attempt a definition of walking which will apply to all cases – at least in a single sentence!

Gait is no easier to define than walking, many dictionaries regarding it as a word primarily for use in connection with horses! This is understandable, since quadruped animals have a repertoire of natural gaits (walking, trotting, cantering, galloping, etc.), as well as some artificial ones, such as that learned by 'Tennessee walking horses' in the area where the author lives. Most people, including the author, tend to use the words gait and walking interchangeably. However, there is a difference: the word gait describes 'the manner or style of walking', rather than the walking process itself. It thus makes more sense to talk about a difference in gait between two individuals than about a difference in walking.

HISTORY

The history of gait analysis has shown a steady progression from early descriptive studies, through increasingly sophisticated methods of measurement, to mathematical analysis and mathematical modeling. Only a brief account of the development of the discipline will be given here. Good reviews of the early years of gait analysis have been given by Garrison (1929), Bresler & Frankel (1950) and Steindler (1953). The more recent history of gait analysis, and of clinical gait analysis in particular, was covered in three excellent review papers by Sutherland (2001, 2002, 2005).

Descriptive studies

Walking has undoubtedly been observed ever since the time of the first men, but the systematic study of gait appears to date from the Renaissance when Leonardo da Vinci, Galileo and Newton all gave useful descriptions of walking. The earliest account using a truly scientific approach was in the classic *De Motu Animalum*, published in 1682 by Borelli, who worked in Italy and was a student of Galileo. Borelli measured the center of gravity of the body and described how balance is maintained in walking by constant forward movement of the supporting area provided by the feet.

The Weber brothers in Germany gave the first clear description of the gait cycle in 1836. They made accurate measurements of the timing of gait and of the pendulum-like swinging of the leg of a cadaver.

Kinematics

Two pioneers of kinematic measurement worked on opposite sides of the Atlantic in the 1870s. Marey, working in Paris, published a study of human limb movements in 1873. He made multiple photographic exposures, on a single plate, of a subject who was dressed in black, except for brightly illuminated stripes on the limbs. He also investigated the path of the center of gravity of the body and the pressure beneath the foot. Eadweard Muybridge (born in England as Edward Muggeridge) became famous in California in 1878 by demonstrating that, when a horse is trotting, there are times when it has all four of its feet off the ground at once. The measurements were made using 24 cameras, triggered in quick succession as the horse ran into thin wires stretched across the track. In the next few years, Muybridge made a further series of studies, of naked human beings walking, running and performing a surprising variety of other activities!

The most serious application of the science of mechanics to human gait during the 19th century was the publication in Germany, in 1895, of *Der Gang des Menschen*, by Braune and Fischer. They employed a technique similar to Marey's, but using fluorescent strip-lights on the limbs instead of white stripes. The resulting photographs were used to determine the three-dimensional trajectories, velocities and accelerations of the body segments. Knowing the masses and accelerations of the body segments, they were then able to estimate the forces involved at all stages during the walking cycle.

Further valuable work on the dynamics of locomotion was done by Bernstein in Moscow in the 1930s. He developed a variety of photographic techniques for kinematic measurement and studied over 150 subjects. Particular attention was paid to the center of gravity of the individual limb segments and of the body as a whole.

Force platforms

Further progress followed the development of the force platform (also called the forceplate). This instrument has contributed greatly to the scientific study of gait and is now standard equipment in gait laboratories. It measures the direction and magnitude of the ground reaction force beneath the foot. An early design was described by Amar in 1924 and an improved one by Elftman in 1938. Both were purely mechanical, the force applied to the platform causing the movement of a pointer. In Elftman's design the pointers were photographed by a high-speed cine camera.

Muscle activity

For a full understanding of normal gait, it is necessary to know which muscles are active during the different parts of the gait cycle. The role of the muscles was studied by Scherb, in Switzerland, during the 1940s, initially by palpating the muscles as his subject walked on a treadmill, then later by the use of electromyography (EMG).

Further advances in the understanding of muscle activity and many other aspects of normal gait were made during the 1940s and 1950s by a very active group working in the University of California at San Francisco and Berkeley, notable among whom was Verne Inman. This group later went on to write *Human Walking* (Inman *et al.*, 1981), published just after Inman's death, which to many people is the definitive textbook on normal gait. After being out of print for some time, a second edition of the book has been published (Rose & Gamble, 1994).

Mechanical analysis

A major contribution to the mechanical analysis of walking, also from the Californian group, was made by Bresler & Frankel (1950). They performed free-body calculations for the hip, knee and ankle joints, allowing for ground reaction forces, the effects of gravity on the limb segments and the inertial forces. The analytical techniques developed by these workers formed the basis of many current methods of modeling and analysis.

An important paper describing the possible mechanisms which the body uses to minimize energy consumption in walking, again from California, was published by Saunders *et al.* (1953). Further important work on energy consumption and in particular the energy transfers between the body segments in walking, was published by Cavagna & Margaria (1966), working in Italy.

By 1960, research began to concentrate on the variability of walking, the development of gait in children and the deterioration of gait in old age. Patricia Murray, working in Milwaukee, Wisconsin, published a series of papers on these subjects, including a detailed review (Murray, 1967).

Mathematical modeling

Once the motions of the body segments and the actions of the different muscles had been examined and documented, attention passed to the forces generated across the joints. Although limited calculations of this type had been made previously, the study by Paul (1965) was the first detailed analysis of hip joint forces during walking. A subsequent paper by the same author also included an analysis of the forces in the knee (Paul, 1966). Since then there have been many mathematical studies of force generation and transmission across the hip, knee and ankle.

The 1970s and 1980s saw great improvements in methods of measurement. The development of more convenient kinematic systems, based on electronics rather than photography, meant that results could be produced in minutes rather than days. Reliable force platforms with a high-frequency response became available, as well as convenient and reliable EMG systems. The availability of high-quality three-dimensional data on the kinetics and kinematics of walking, and the ease of access to powerful computers, made it possible to develop increasingly sophisticated mathematical models. Gait laboratories now routinely measure joint moments and powers for the hip, knee and ankle. Somewhat less reliably, estimates can also be made of muscle, ligament and joint contact forces.

Clinical application

From the earliest days, it has been the hope of most of those working in this field that gait measurements would be found useful in the management of patients with walking disorders. Many of the early workers made studies of people who walked with abnormal gait patterns and some (notably Amar, Scherb and the Californian group) attempted to use the results for the benefit of individual patients. However, the results were not particularly impressive.

Since 1960, there has been a more serious attempt to take gait analysis out of the research laboratory and into the clinic. With the improvements in measurement and analytical techniques, the major limitation now is not the ability to produce high-quality data but knowing how best to use these data for the benefit of patients. It is fair to say that in the early days, far more progress was made in scientific gait analysis, particularly as applied to normal subjects, than in the application of these techniques for the benefit of those with gait disorders. However, since about 1980, there has been a steady increase in the effective use of gait analysis in the clinical management of patients.

As well as a gradual increase in the clinical use of scientific gait analysis, there has also been a growing interest in the use of observational or visual gait analysis. This has become much easier to perform since video cameras and video cassette recorders (VCRs) have become widely available.

As stated above, the history of clinical gait analysis was reviewed by Sutherland (2001, 2002, 2005).

TERMINOLOGY USED IN GAIT ANALYSIS

The *gait cycle* is defined as the time interval between two successive occurrences of one of the repetitive events of walking. Although any event could be chosen to define the gait cycle, it is generally convenient to use the instant at which one foot contacts the ground ('initial contact'). If it is decided to start with initial contact of the right foot, as shown in Fig. 2.1, then the cycle will continue until the right foot contacts the ground again. The left foot, of course, goes through exactly the same series of events as the right, but displaced in time by half a cycle.

The following terms are used to identify major events during the gait cycle:

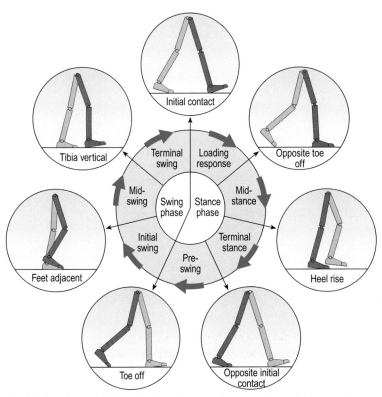

Fig. 2.1 Positions of the legs during a single gait cycle by the right leg (gray).

1. Initial contact
2. Opposite toe off
3. Heel rise
4. Opposite initial contact
5. Toe off
6. Feet adjacent
7. Tibia vertical
(1. Initial contact).

These seven events subdivide the gait cycle into seven periods, four of which occur in the stance phase, when the foot is on the ground, and three in the swing phase, when the foot is moving forward through the air (Fig. 2.1). The stance phase, which is also called the 'support phase' or 'contact phase', lasts from initial contact to toe off. It is subdivided into:

1. Loading response
2. Mid-stance
3. Terminal stance
4. Pre-swing.

The swing phase lasts from toe off to the next initial contact. It is subdivided into:

1. Initial swing
2. Mid-swing
3. Terminal swing.

The duration of a complete gait cycle is known as the *cycle time*, which is divided into *stance time* and *swing time*.

Unfortunately, the nomenclature used to describe the gait cycle varies considerably from one publication to another. The present text attempts to use terms which will be understood by most people working in the field; alternative terminology will be given where appropriate. Wall *et al.* (1987) pointed out that the usual terminology is inadequate to describe some severely pathological gaits.

Gait cycle timing

Figure 2.2 shows the timings of initial contact and toe off for both feet during a little more than one gait cycle. Right initial contact occurs while the left foot is still on the ground and there is a period of *double support* (also known as 'double limb stance') between initial contact on the right and toe off on the left. During the swing phase on the left side, only the right foot is on the

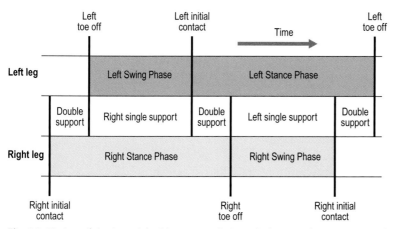

Fig. 2.2 Timing of single and double support during a little more than one gait cycle, starting with right initial contact.

ground, giving a period of *right single support* (or 'single limb stance'), which ends with initial contact by the left foot. There is then another period of double support, until toe off on the right side. *Left single support* corresponds to the right swing phase and the cycle ends with the next initial contact on the right.

In each double support phase, one foot is forward, having just landed on the ground, and the other one is backward, being just about to leave the ground. When it is necessary to distinguish between the two legs in the double support phase, the leg in front is usually known as the 'leading' leg and the leg behind as the 'trailing' leg. The leading leg is in 'loading response', sometimes referred to as 'braking double support', 'initial double support' or 'weight acceptance'. The trailing leg is in 'pre-swing', also known as 'second', 'terminal' or 'thrusting' double support or 'weight release'.

In each gait cycle, there are thus two periods of double support and two periods of single support. The stance phase usually lasts about 60% of the cycle, the swing phase about 40% and each period of double support about 10%. However, this varies with the speed of walking, the swing phase becoming proportionally longer and the stance phase and double support phases shorter, as the speed increases (Murray, 1967). The final disappearance of the double support phase marks the transition from walking to running. Between successive steps in running there is a *flight phase*, also known as the 'float', 'double-float' or 'non-support' phase, when neither foot is on the ground. A detailed study of gait cycle timing was published by Blanc *et al.* (1999).

Foot placement

The terms used to describe the placement of the feet on the ground are shown in Fig. 2.3. The *stride length* is the distance between two successive placements

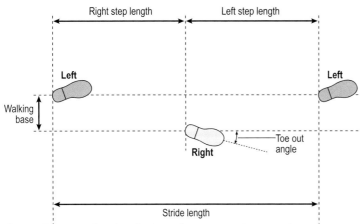

Fig. 2.3 Terms used to describe foot placement on the ground.

of the same foot. It consists of two *step lengths*, left and right, each of which is the distance by which the named foot moves forward in front of the other one. In pathological gait, it is common for the two step lengths to be different. If the left foot is moved forward to take a step and the right one is brought up beside it, rather than in front of it, the right step length will be zero. It is even possible for the step length on one side to be negative, if that foot never catches up with the other one. However, the *stride* length, measured between successive positions of the left foot, must always be the same as the stride length measured between successive positions of the right foot, unless the subject is walking around a curve.

This definition of a 'stride', consisting of one 'step' by each foot, breaks down in some pathological gaits, in which one foot makes a series of 'hopping' movements while the other is in the air (Wall *et al.*, 1987). There is no satisfactory nomenclature to deal with this situation.

The *walking base* (also known as the 'stride width' or 'base of support') is the side-to-side distance between the line of the two feet, usually measured at the midpoint of the back of the heel but sometimes below the center of the ankle joint. The preferred units for stride length and step length are meters and for the walking base, millimeters. The pattern of walking known as 'tandem gait' involves walking with the heel of one foot placed directly in front of the toes of the other, i.e. with a walking base close to zero. Although this pattern is not typically seen, even as a pathological gait, it requires good balance and coordination and it is often used by the police as a test for intoxication!

The *toe out* (or, less commonly, *toe in*) is the angle in degrees between the direction of progression and a reference line on the sole of the foot. The reference line varies from one study to another; it may be defined anatomically but is commonly the midline of the foot, as judged by eye.

It is common experience that you need to walk more carefully on ice than on asphalt. Whether or not the foot slips during walking depends on two things: the coefficient of friction between the foot and the ground, and the relationship between the vertical force and the forces parallel to the walking surface (front-to-back and side-to-side). The ratio of the horizontal to the vertical force is known as the 'utilized coefficient of friction' and slippage will occur if this exceeds the actual coefficient of friction between the foot and the ground. In normal walking, a coefficient of friction of 0.35–0.40 is generally sufficient to prevent slippage; the most hazardous part of the gait cycle for slippage is initial contact. There is a fairly extensive literature on foot-to-ground friction and slippage, e.g. Cham & Redfern (2002) and Burnfield *et al.* (2005).

Cadence, cycle time and speed

The *cadence* is the number of steps taken in a given time, the usual units being steps per minute. In most other types of scientific measurement, complete cycles are counted, but as there are two steps in a single gait cycle, the cadence is a measure of half-cycles. Measurement in 'steps per minute' does not conform with the Système International (SI). A scientifically acceptable alternative would be to measure cadence in steps per second, but there is currently a trend to replace cadence entirely by a quantity which is inversely related to it – the *cycle time*, also known as the 'stride time', in seconds:

cycle time (s) = 120/cadence (steps/min)

The normal ranges for both cadence and cycle time in both sexes at different ages are given in Appendix 1.

The *speed* of walking is the distance covered by the whole body in a given time. It should be measured in meters per second. Many authors use the term 'velocity' in place of 'speed' but this is an incorrect usage of the term, unless the direction of walking is also stated, since velocity is a vector. The instantaneous speed varies from one instant to another during the walking cycle, but the average speed is the product of the cadence and the stride length, providing appropriate units are used. The cadence, in steps per minute, corresponds to half-strides per 60 seconds or full strides per 120 seconds. The speed can thus be calculated from cadence and stride length using the formula:

speed (m/s) = stride length (m) × cadence (steps/min)/120

If cycle time is used in place of cadence, the calculation becomes much more straightforward:

speed (m/s) = stride length (m)/cycle time (s)

The walking speed thus depends on the two step lengths, which in turn depend to a large extent on the duration of the swing phase on each side. The step length is the amount by which the foot can be moved forwards during the swing phase, so that a short swing phase on one side will generally reduce the step length on that side. If the foot catches on the ground, this may terminate the swing phase and thereby further reduce both step length and walking speed. In pathological gait, the step length is often shortened, but it behaves in a way which is counterintuitive. When pathology affects one foot more than the other, an individual will usually try to spend a shorter time on the 'bad' foot and correspondingly longer on the 'good' one. Shortening the stance phase on the 'bad' foot means bringing the 'good' foot to the ground sooner, thereby shortening both the duration of the swing phase and the step length on that side. Thus, a short step length on one side generally means problems with single support on the *other* side.

When making comparisons between individuals, particularly with children, it is useful to allow for differences in size. This is done by dividing a measurement by some aspect of body size, such as height (stature) or leg length, a procedure generally known as 'normalization'. It is thus fairly common to see walking speed expressed in 'statures per second' or to see measures such as 'step factor', which is step length divided by leg length (Sutherland, 1997).

Since walking speed depends on both cadence and stride length, it follows that speed may be changed by altering only one of these variables, for instance by increasing the cadence while keeping the stride length constant. In practice, however, people normally change their walking speed by adjusting both cadence and stride length. Sekiya & Nagasaki (1998) defined the 'walk ratio' as step length (m) divided by step rate (steps/min) and found that it was fairly constant in both males and females over a range of walking speeds from very slow to very fast. Macellari *et al.* (1999) made a detailed study of the relationships between gender, body size, walking speed, gait timing and foot placement.

OUTLINE OF THE GAIT CYCLE

The purpose of this section is to provide the reader with an overview of the gait cycle, to make the detailed description which follows a little easier to follow. The cycle is illustrated by Figs 2.4–2.8 and 2.10–2.20, all of which are taken from a single walk by a 22-year-old normal female, weight 540 N (55 kgf, 121 lbf), walking barefoot with a cycle time of 0.88 s (cadence 136 steps/min), a stride length of 1.50 m and a speed of 1.70 m/s. The individual measurements from this subject do not always correspond to 'average' values, because of the normal variability between individuals, although they are all close to the normal range. The measurements were all made in the plane of progression, which is a vertical plane aligned to the direction of the walk; in normal walking it closely corresponds to the sagittal plane of the body. The data were obtained using a Vicon television/computer system and a Bertec force platform. It should be noted that different laboratories use different methods of measurement, so that other publications may quote different values for some of the measured variables. The reader should thus concentrate on the changes in the variables during the gait cycle, rather than on their absolute values.

When examining diagrams of the joint angles through the gait cycle, it is essential to understand how the angles are defined. Generally speaking, the knee angle is defined as the angle between the femur and the tibia and there is usually no ambiguity. The ankle angle is usually defined as the angle between the tibia and an arbitrary line in the foot. Although this angle is normally around 90°, it is conventional to define it as 0°, dorsiflexion and plantarflexion being movements in the positive and negative directions. In this book, dorsiflexion is a positive angle, but in some other publications it is negative. The 'hip' angle may be measured in two different ways: the angle between the vertical and the femur, and the angle between the pelvis and the femur. The latter is the 'true' hip angle and is usually defined so that 0° is close to the hip angle in the standing position. Forward flexion of the trunk appears as hip flexion when the hip angle is defined with reference to the pelvis, but not when it is defined with reference to the vertical.

The descriptions which follow assume that symmetry is present between the two sides of the body. This is approximately true for normal individuals, although detailed examination shows that everyone has some degree of asymmetry (Sadeghi, 2003). Such subtle asymmetries are negligible, however, when contrasted with the majority of pathological gaits.

Some gait studies are performed barefoot and some with the subject wearing shoes. Oeffinger et al. (1999) found small differences in some of the gait parameters between these two conditions in children, but did not consider them to be clinically significant. It is usually at the discretion of the investigator whether or not shoes are worn, although in some cases (e.g. when an ankle–foot orthosis or an orthotic insole is used) this may be dictated by the subject's condition.

During gait, important movements occur in all three planes – sagittal, frontal and transverse. However, this introductory text will concentrate on the sagittal plane, in which the largest movements occur. For information on the motion in other planes, the reader is referred to more detailed texts, such as Perry (1992), Inman et al. (1981) or Rose & Gamble (1994).

Figure 2.4 shows the successive positions of the right leg at 40 ms intervals, measured over a single gait cycle. Figure 2.5 shows the corresponding sagittal plane angles at the hip, knee and ankle joints. Figure 2.6 shows the joint moments (in newton-meters per kilogram body mass) and Fig. 2.7 the joint powers (in watts per kilogram body mass). Different authors have used different units for the measurement of moments and powers; those used here

and efficiency of walking depend to some extent on the motions of the trunk and arms, but these movements are commonly ignored in clinical gait analysis and have been relatively neglected in gait research. The whole trunk rises and falls twice during the cycle, through a total range of about 46 mm (Perry, 1992), being lowest during double support and highest in the middle of the stance and swing phases. An approximation to this vertical motion can be seen in the position of the hip joint in Fig. 2.4. The trunk also moves from side to side, once in each cycle, the trunk being over each leg during its stance phase, as might be expected from the need for support. The total range of side-to-side movement is also about 46 mm (Perry, 1992). The pelvis, as well as twisting about a vertical axis, also tips slightly, both backwards and forwards (with an associated change in lumbar lordosis) and from side to side. The spinal muscles are selectively activated so that the head moves less than the pelvis, which is important for providing a stable platform for vision (Prince *et al.*, 1994).

Hip: The hip flexes and extends once during the cycle (Fig. 2.5). The limit of flexion is reached around the middle of the swing phase and the hip is then kept flexed until initial contact. The peak extension is reached before the end of the stance phase, after which the hip begins to flex again.

Knee: The knee shows two flexion and two extension peaks during each gait cycle. It is more or less fully extended before initial contact, flexes during the loading response and the early part of mid-stance ('stance phase knee flexion'), extends again during the later part of mid-stance, then starts flexing again, reaching a peak during initial swing ('swing phase knee flexion'). It extends again prior to the next initial contact.

Ankle and foot: The ankle is usually within a few degrees of the neutral position for dorsiflexion/plantarflexion at the time of initial contact. After initial contact, the ankle plantarflexes, bringing the forefoot down onto the ground. During mid-stance, the tibia moves forward over the foot, and the ankle joint becomes dorsiflexed. Before opposite initial contact, the ankle angle again changes, a major plantarflexion taking place until just after toe off. During the swing phase, the ankle moves back into dorsiflexion until the forefoot has cleared the ground (around feet adjacent), after which something close to the neutral position is maintained until the next initial contact. In the frontal plane, the foot is slightly inverted (supinated, adducted or varus) at initial contact. The foot pronates as it contacts the ground, then moves back into supination as the ankle angle changes from plantarflexion to dorsiflexion, this supinated attitude being maintained as the heel rises and the ankle plantarflexes prior to toe off. Some degree of supination is retained throughout the swing phase.

THE GAIT CYCLE IN DETAIL

Each of the following sections begins with some general remarks about the events surrounding a particular event in the gait cycle and then describes what is happening in the upper body, hips, knees, ankles and feet, with particular reference to the activity of the muscles. These sections are very detailed and may be too much to comprehend in one 'pass'. It is suggested that the reader should skip the moments and powers on the first reading, but should go back to them later, to gain a deeper understanding of the mechanical processes underlying the gait cycle.

More detailed descriptions of the events of normal gait are given by Murray (1967), Perry (1992), Inman *et al.* (1981) and Rose & Gamble (1994).

Initial contact (Fig. 2.10)

1. General: Initial contact is the beginning of the loading response, which is the first period of the stance phase. Initial contact is frequently called 'heelstrike', since in normal individuals there is often a distinct impact between the heel and the ground, known as the 'heelstrike transient'. Other names for this event are 'heel contact', 'footstrike' or 'foot contact'. The direction of the ground reaction force changes from generally upwards during the heelstrike transient (Fig. 2.10) to upwards and backwards in the loading

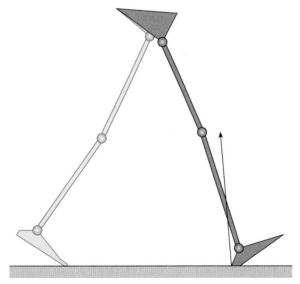

Fig. 2.10 Initial contact: position of right leg (gray), left leg (blue) and ground reaction force vector during the heelstrike transient. This illustration also applies to terminal foot contact.

response, immediately afterwards (Fig. 2.11). This change in direction can also be seen in the butterfly diagram (Fig. 2.8), where the force vector changes direction immediately after initial contact.

2. Upper body: The trunk is about half a stride length behind the leading (right) foot at the time of initial contact. In the side-to-side direction, the trunk is crossing the midline in its range of travel, moving towards the right, as the foot on that side makes contact. The trunk is twisted, the left shoulder and the right side of the pelvis each being at their furthest forwards and the left arm at its most advanced. The amount of arm swinging varies greatly from one person to another and it also increases with the speed of walking. At the time of initial contact, Murray (1967) found the mean elbow flexion was 8° and the shoulder flexion 45°.

3. Hip: The attitude of the legs at the time of initial contact is shown in Fig. 2.10. The maximum flexion of the hip (generally around 30°) is reached around the middle of the swing phase, after which it changes little until initial contact. The hamstrings are active during the latter part of the swing phase (since they act to prevent knee hyperextension); gluteus maximus begins to contract around the time of initial contact and together these muscles start the extension of the hip, which will be complete around the time of opposite initial contact (Fig. 2.5).

4. Knee: The knee extends rapidly at the end of the swing phase, becoming more or less straight just before initial contact and then starting to flex again

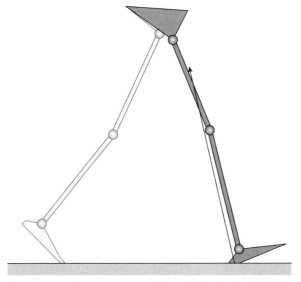

Fig. 2.11 Loading response: position of right leg (gray), left leg (blue) and ground reaction force vector 20 ms after initial contact.

(Figs 2.5 and 2.10). This extension is generally thought to be passive, although Perry (1992) states that it involves quadriceps contraction. Except in very slow walking, the hamstrings contract eccentrically at the end of the swing phase, to act as a braking mechanism to prevent knee hyperextension. This contraction continues into the beginning of the stance phase.

5. Ankle and foot: The ankle is generally close to its neutral position in plantarflexion/dorsiflexion at the time of initial contact. Since the tibia is sloping backwards, the foot slopes upwards and only the heel contacts the ground (Fig. 2.10). The foot is usually slightly supinated (inverted, adducted or varus) at this time and most people show a wear pattern on the lateral side of the heel of the shoe. Tibialis anterior is active throughout swing and in early stance, having maintained dorsiflexion during the swing phase and in preparation for the controlled movement into plantarflexion which occurs following initial contact.

6. Moments and powers: At the time of initial contact, there is an internal extensor moment at the hip (Fig. 2.6), produced by contraction of the hip extensors (gluteus maximus and the hamstrings, Fig. 2.9). As the hip joint moves in the direction of extension, these muscles contract concentrically and generate power (H1 in Fig. 2.7). The knee shows an internal flexor moment, due to contraction of the hamstrings (Fig. 2.9) as they prevent hyperextension at the end of the swing phase. As the knee starts to flex, concentric contraction of the hamstrings, as well as the release of energy stored in the ligaments of the extended knee, results in a short-lived power generation (unnamed peak in Fig. 2.7). Little moment or power exchange occurs at the ankle until just after initial contact. The 'heelstrike' involves an absorption of energy by the elastic tissues of the heel and by compliant materials in footwear, very little of which could be recovered later in the stance phase. The amount of energy lost to the environment as sound and heat in this way is probably fairly small.

Loading response (Fig. 2.11)

1. General: The loading response is the double support period between initial contact and opposite toe off. During this period, the foot is lowered to the ground by plantarflexion of the ankle. The ground reaction force increases rapidly in magnitude, its direction being upwards and backwards. In the subject used for illustration, loading response occupied the period from 0% to 7% of the cycle; this is unusually short, loading response typically occupying the first 10–12% of the cycle. Fig. 2.11 represents 2% of the cycle.

2. Upper body: During loading response, the trunk is at its lowest vertical position, about 20 mm below its average level for the whole cycle; its instantaneous forward speed is at its greatest, around 10% higher than the average speed for the whole cycle. It continues to move laterally towards the right foot. The arms, having reached their maximum forward (left) and backward (right) positions, begin to return.

3. Hip: During loading response, the hip begins to extend (Fig. 2.5), through concentric contraction of the hip extensors, gluteus maximus and the hamstrings (Fig. 2.9).

4. Knee: From its nearly fully extended position at initial contact, the knee flexes during loading response (Fig. 2.5), initiating the 'stance phase flexion'. This is accompanied by eccentric contraction of the quadriceps (Fig. 2.9), to limit the speed and magnitude of flexion.

5. Ankle and foot: The loading response period of the gait cycle, also called the 'initial rocker', 'heel rocker' or 'heel pivot', involves plantarflexion at the ankle (Fig. 2.5). The plantarflexion is permitted by eccentric contraction of the tibialis anterior muscle. The movement into plantarflexion is accompanied by pronation of the foot and internal rotation of the tibia, there being an automatic coupling between pronation/supination of the foot and internal/external rotation of the tibia (Inman et al., 1981; Rose & Gamble, 1994). The direction of the force vector changes from that shown in Fig. 2.10 to that shown in Fig. 2.11, within 10–20 ms.

6. Moments and powers: As described above (p. 66, initial contact, section 6), the hip shows an internal extensor moment with power generation during the loading response and the knee shows an internal flexor moment with power generation. At the ankle, the posterior placement of the force vector (Fig. 2.11) produces an external plantarflexor moment. In the normal individual, this is resisted by an internal dorsiflexor moment (Fig. 2.6) produced by tibialis anterior (Fig. 2.9), which contracts eccentrically, absorbing power (Fig. 2.7) and permitting the foot to be lowered gently to the ground. Should tibialis anterior fail to generate sufficient moment, the foot dorsiflexes too rapidly, producing an audible 'foot slap'.

Opposite toe off (Fig. 2.12)

1. General: Opposite toe off, also known as 'opposite foot off', is the end of the double support period known as loading response and the beginning of mid-stance, the first period of single support. The forefoot, which was being

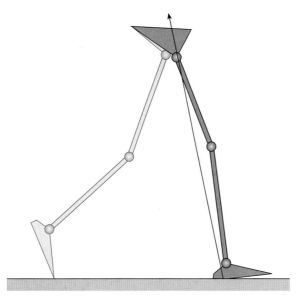

Fig. 2.12 Opposite toe off: position of right leg (gray), left leg (blue) and ground reaction force vector.

lowered by plantarflexion of the ankle, contacts the ground at 'foot flat', also known as 'forefoot contact', which generally occurs around the time of opposite toe off. On the opposite (left) side, it marks the end of the stance phase and the beginning of the swing phase. In the subject used for illustration, opposite toe off (Fig. 2.12) occurred at 7% of the cycle and foot flat at 8% of the cycle.

2. Upper body: At opposite toe off, the left shoulder and arm, having reached their most advanced position, are now moving back again. Similarly, the pelvis on the right side now starts to twist back towards the neutral position. The trunk, having reached its lowest position during loading response, now begins to gain height but to lose forward speed, as a result of the backward and upward direction of the ground reaction force, acting on the center of gravity of the body. This represents a conversion of kinetic energy to potential energy, similar to that seen in a child's swing.

3. Hip: The hip flexion angle is around 25° at time of opposite toe off (Fig. 2.5). The hip continues to extend, by concentric contraction of the gluteus maximus and hamstrings.

4. Knee: At opposite toe off, the knee is continuing to flex, reaching the peak of 'stance phase knee flexion' early in mid-stance, after which it begins to extend again (Fig. 2.5). The magnitude of the stance phase flexion is very sensitive to walking speed; it disappears in a very slow walk. Quadriceps contraction (eccentric then concentric) permits the knee to act like a spring, preventing the vertical force from building up too rapidly (Perry, 1974).

5. Ankle and foot: As soon as the foot is flat on the ground, around opposite toe off, the direction of ankle motion changes from plantarflexion to dorsiflexion, as the tibia moves over the now stationary foot (Fig. 2.5). Both foot pronation and internal tibial rotation reach a peak around opposite toe off and begin to reverse. These two motions are 'coupled', i.e. they always occur together, due in part to the geometry of the ankle and subtalar joints (Inman et al., 1981; Rose & Gamble, 1994). Tibialis anterior ceases to contract, to be replaced by contraction of the triceps surae (Fig. 2.9).

6. Moments and powers: At opposite toe off, the hip continues to have an internal extensor moment with power generation, as described above (p. 66, initial contact, section 6). At the knee, the force vector lies behind the joint (Fig. 2.12), producing an external flexor moment. This is opposed by an internal extensor moment (Fig. 2.6), generated by the quadriceps muscles (Fig. 2.9). These contract eccentrically, absorbing power (K1 in Fig. 2.7). The line of the ground reaction force begins to move forwards along the foot (Fig. 2.12), causing the internal dorsiflexor moment at the ankle to become smaller and then to reverse, to become a plantarflexor moment (Fig. 2.6). Little power exchange occurs at the ankle at this time.

Mid-stance (Fig. 2.13)

1. General: Mid-stance is the period of the gait cycle between opposite toe off and heel rise, although the term has been used in the past to describe an event

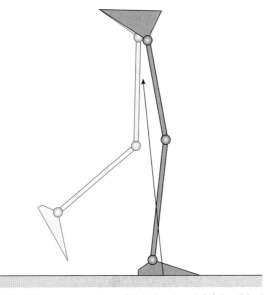

Fig. 2.13 Mid-stance: position of right leg (gray), left leg (blue) and ground reaction force vector 100 ms after opposite toe off.

of the gait cycle – the time at which the swing phase leg passes the stance phase leg, corresponding to the swing phase event of 'feet adjacent'. In the subject used for illustration, mid-stance occupied the period from 7% to 32% of the cycle; Fig. 2.13 represents 18% of the cycle.

2. Upper body: The period of mid-stance sees the trunk climbing to its highest point, about 20 mm above the mean level, and slowing its forward speed, as the kinetic energy of forward motion is converted to the potential energy of height. The side-to-side motion of the trunk also reaches its peak during mid-stance, the trunk being displaced about 20 mm from its central position, towards the side of the stance (right) leg. Like the feet, the arms pass each other during mid-stance, as each follows the motion of the opposite leg. The twisting of the trunk has now disappeared, as both the shoulder girdle and pelvis pass through neutral before twisting the other way.

3. Hip: During the mid-stance period, the hip continues to extend, moving from a flexed attitude to an extended one (Fig. 2.5). Concentric contraction of gluteus maximus and the hamstrings ceases during this period, as hip extension is achieved by inertia and gravity. Throughout mid-stance and terminal stance, significant muscle activity about the hip joint takes place in the frontal plane. As soon as the opposite foot has left the ground, the pelvis is supported only by the stance phase hip. It is permitted to dip down slightly on the side of the swinging leg, but its position is maintained by contraction of the hip abductors, especially gluteus medius and tensor fascia lata.

4. Knee: During mid-stance, the knee reaches its peak of stance phase flexion and starts to extend again (Fig. 2.5), initially through concentric contraction of the quadriceps. The peak generally occurs at between 15% and 20% of the gait cycle. Its magnitude is variable, both from one individual to another and with the speed of walking, but it is commonly between 10° and 20°.

5. Ankle and foot: The 'mid-stance rocker', also called the 'second rocker' or 'ankle rocker', occurs during mid-stance and terminal stance. It is characterized by forward rotation of the tibia about the ankle joint, as the foot remains flat on the floor, the ankle angle changing from plantarflexion to dorsiflexion, with the triceps surae contracting eccentrically. The actual angles vary with the method of measurement; most authors report larger angles than those seen in Fig. 2.5. External rotation of the tibia and coupled supination of the foot occur during mid-stance and terminal stance. The ground reaction force vector moves forward along the foot from the time of foot flat onwards, moving into the forefoot prior to heel rise. The movement of the foot into supination peaks in mid-stance and then begins to reverse towards pronation.

6. Moments and powers: During mid-stance, the internal extensor moment at the hip, generated by contraction of the extensor muscles, declines and disappears, to be replaced by a moment in the opposite direction (Fig. 2.6). At the knee, the force vector remains behind the joint, producing an external flexor moment, opposed by an internal extensor moment (Fig. 2.6), due to quadriceps contraction (Fig. 2.9). According to Perry (1992), only the vasti, and not the rectus femoris, are active at this time. As the direction of knee motion changes from flexion to extension (Fig. 2.5), power generation takes place (K2 in Fig. 2.6). The ankle shows an increasing internal plantarflexor moment throughout mid-stance and into terminal stance (Fig. 2.6), as the force vector moves into the forefoot. This moment is generated by the triceps surae (Fig. 2.9), contracting eccentrically and absorbing power (A1 in Fig. 2.7).

Heel rise (Fig. 2.14)

1. General: Heel rise, also called 'heel off', marks the transition from mid-stance to terminal stance. It is the time at which the heel begins to lift from the walking surface. Its timing varies considerably, both from one individual to another and with the speed of walking. The subject used for illustration showed heel rise at 32% of the gait cycle.

2. Upper body: By heel rise, the trunk is falling from its highest point, reached during mid-stance. The lateral displacement over the supporting

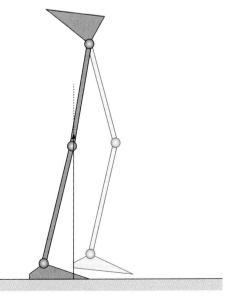

Fig. 2.14 Heel rise: position of right leg (gray), left leg (blue) and ground reaction force vector.

(right) leg also begins to diminish, in preparation for the transfer of weight back to the left leg. As the right hip extends and the leg moves backwards, the right side of the pelvis twists backwards with it and the arm and shoulder girdle on the right move forwards.

3. Hip: At heel rise and into terminal stance, the hip continues to extend (Fig. 2.5). Peak hip extension is reached around the time of opposite initial contact. The activity of the hip abductors in the frontal plane is still required to stabilize the pelvis, although this activity ceases prior to initial contact by the other foot.

4. Knee: The knee has an extension peak close to the time of heel rise (Fig. 2.5). Around this time, active ankle plantarflexion brings the ground reaction force forward, moving it into the forefoot and in front of the knee joint (barely visible in Fig. 2.14). This attempts to extend the knee, an effect known as the 'plantarflexion/knee extension couple', which becomes very important in some pathological gaits. Contraction of the gastrocnemius augments the action of the soleus as far as the ankle joint is concerned, but it also acts as a flexor at the knee, preventing hyperextension and subsequently initiating knee flexion.

5. Ankle and foot: The peak of ankle dorsiflexion is reached some time after heel rise (Fig. 2.5). Triceps surae initially maintains the ankle angle as the knee begins to flex, with movement into plantarflexion only beginning late in terminal stance. The tibia becomes increasingly externally rotated and the foot becomes increasingly supinated, the two being linked through coupled motion at the subtalar joint. As the heel rises, the toes remain flat on the ground and extension occurs at the metatarsophalangeal (MTP) joints, along an oblique line across the foot, known as the 'metatarsal break' or 'toe break'. From the time that the heel rises, hindfoot inversion (adduction or varus angulation) is seen.

6. Moments and powers: At heel rise there is a small but increasing internal hip flexor moment (Fig. 2.6). The source of this internal flexor moment does not appear to have been fully explained in the literature, although it could be due to a combination of adductor longus and rectus femoris contraction and stretching of ligaments as the hip moves into extension, with a resulting power absorption (H2 in Fig. 2.7). At the knee, quadriceps contraction has ceased prior to heel rise and the internal knee moment has reversed to become flexor. According to Perry (1992), this occurs because the upper body moves forward faster than the tibia. If the ankle joint were totally free, the forward motion of the body would simply dorsiflex the ankle. However, contraction of the triceps surae (Fig. 2.9) slows down the forward motion of the tibia so that as the femur moves forwards, an external extensor moment is generated at the knee, opposed by an internal flexor moment (Fig. 2.6). Only small and variable power exchanges occur at the knee around heel rise. At the ankle, the internal dorsiflexor moment continues to increase, as first the soleus and then both soleus and gastrocnemius together (triceps surae in Fig. 2.9) contract increasingly strongly. The contraction is initially eccentric, with power absorption (A1 in Fig. 2.7).

Opposite initial contact (Fig. 2.15)

1. General: As might be expected, opposite initial contact in symmetrical gait occurs at close to 50% of the cycle. It marks the end of the period of single support and the beginning of pre-swing, which is the second period of double support. At the time of opposite initial contact, also known as 'opposite foot contact', the hip begins to flex, the knee is already flexing and the ankle is plantarflexing. The period between heel rise and toe off (terminal stance followed by pre-swing) is sometimes called the 'terminal rocker'. This is appropriate, since the leg is now rotating forwards about the forefoot, rather than about the ankle joint. Another term for this period is the 'push off' phase. Perry (1974) objected to this term, suggesting instead the term 'roll-off', because 'the late floor-reaction peak is the result of leverage by body alignment, rather than an active downward thrust'. However, it is clear that the 'push off' is not simply passive, since it is the period during which the generation of power at the ankle is greatest (Winter, 1983). What is not clear is whether this power is used to accelerate the whole body (as suggested by

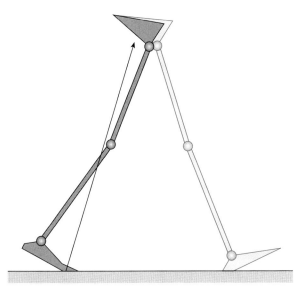

Fig. 2.15 Opposite initial contact: position of right leg (gray), left leg (blue) and ground reaction force vector.

Winter) or merely the leg (as suggested by Perry) or (as seems most likely) some combination of the two. Buczek *et al.* (2003) showed that power generation at the ankle is necessary to sustain normal walking. Using terms borrowed from the study of posture control, normal walking involves an 'ankle strategy' but may be replaced by a 'hip strategy' in which subjects 'decrease their push-off, pulling their leg forward from their hips' (Mueller *et al.*, 1994).

2. Upper body: The attitude of the upper body at opposite initial contact resembles that described for initial contact, except that the trunk is now moving towards the left rather than the right and the trunk is twisted so that the right shoulder and arm and the left side of the pelvis are forward.

3. Hip: At opposite initial contact, the hip reaches its most extended position (typically between 10° and 20° of extension, depending on how it is measured) and motion reverses in the direction of flexion (Fig 2.5). With the hip extended, adductor longus acts as the primary hip flexor (Perry, 1992) and probably generates sufficient moment to initiate hip flexion, particularly when combined with tension in the stretched hip ligaments and the effects of gravity.

4. Knee: The knee is already moving into flexion by the time of opposite initial contact (Fig. 2.5). The force vector has moved behind the knee, aiding its flexion (Fig. 2.15) and rectus femoris begins to contract eccentrically (included with quadriceps in Fig. 2.9), to prevent flexion from occurring too rapidly. The term 'pull off' has been used for the hip and knee flexion which occur during pre-swing.

5. Ankle and foot: From before opposite initial contact until the foot leaves the ground at toe off, the ankle is moving into plantarflexion (Fig. 2.5), due to concentric contraction of the triceps surae (Fig. 2.9). Extension of the toes at the MTP joints continues and causes a tightening of the plantar fascia. The foot reaches its maximal supination, with hindfoot inversion (adduction or varus angulation) and coupled external tibial rotation. These various factors combine to lock the midtarsal joints, resulting in high stability of the foot for loadbearing (Inman *et al.*, 1981; Rose & Gamble, 1994).

6. Moments and powers: A peak of hip internal flexor moment occurs around opposite initial contact (Fig. 2.6). As stated above (p. 74, opposite initial contact, section 3), it probably results from a combination of adductor longus contraction, passive tension in the hip ligaments and gravity. As the direction of hip motion reverses from extension to flexion, power absorption (H2 in Fig. 2.7) is replaced by power generation (H3 in Fig. 2.7). During terminal stance, flexion of the knee brings the joint in front of the force vector (Fig. 2.15), reversing the external moment from extensor to flexor and hence changing the internal moment from flexor to extensor (Fig. 2.6). Eccentric contraction of rectus femoris (included with quadriceps in Fig. 2.9) limits the rate of knee flexion and results in power absorption (K3 in Fig. 2.7). At the ankle, the force vector is well in front of the joint at opposite initial contact (Fig. 2.15). The resulting high external dorsiflexor moment is opposed by a correspondingly high internal plantarflexor moment (Fig. 2.6), produced by concentric contraction of the triceps surae (Fig. 2.9). The result is a large generation of power (A2 in Fig. 2.7), which is the highest power generation of the entire gait cycle. The immediate effect of this power generation is to accelerate the limb forward into the swing phase.

Toe off (Fig. 2.16)

1. General: Toe off generally occurs at about 60% percent of the gait cycle (57% in the subject used for illustration). It separates pre-swing from initial swing and is the point at which the stance phase ends and the swing phase begins. The name 'terminal contact' has been proposed for this event, since in pathological gait the toe may not be the last part of the foot to leave the ground.

2. Upper body: The extreme rotations of the shoulders, arms and trunk all begin to return towards the neutral position, as the trunk gains height and moves towards the new (left) supporting foot.

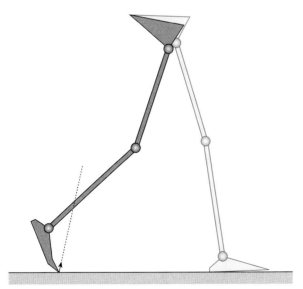

Fig. 2.16 Toe off: position of right leg (gray), left leg (blue) and ground reaction force vector.

3. Hip: As the foot leaves the ground, the hip continues to flex (Fig. 2.5). This is achieved by gravity and tension in the hip ligaments, as well as by contraction of the rectus femoris (included with quadriceps in Fig. 2.9) and adductor longus.

4. Knee: By the time of toe off, the knee has flexed to around half of the angle it will achieve at the peak of swing phase flexion. This flexion is aided by the positioning of the ground reaction force vector well behind the knee (Fig. 2.16), although the magnitude of the force declines rapidly, reaching zero as the foot leaves the ground. The major part of knee flexion then results from hip flexion: the leg acts as a jointed 'double pendulum' so that as the hip flexes, the shank is 'left behind', due to its inertia, resulting in flexion of the knee. At the very beginning of the swing phase, rectus femoris may contract eccentrically to prevent excessive knee flexion, particularly at faster walking speeds (Nene et al., 1999).

5. Ankle and foot: The peak of ankle plantarflexion occurs just after toe off. The magnitude of plantarflexion depends on the method of measurement; it is 25° in Fig. 2.5. Triceps surae contraction ceases prior to toe off and tibialis anterior begins to contract (Fig. 2.9), to bring the ankle up into a neutral or dorsiflexed attitude during the swing phase.

6. Moments and powers: Around toe off, the hip still shows an internal flexor moment (Fig. 2.6), resulting from gravity, ligament elasticity, adductor longus and iliopsoas contraction. Since the hip is flexing at this time, power generation occurs (H3 in Fig. 2.7). As stated above (p. 76, toe off, section 4), during pre-swing and initial swing, hip flexion causes the knee to flex, the 'double pendulum' resulting in an external flexor moment at the knee, opposed by an internal extensor moment (Fig. 2.6), as rectus femoris contracts eccentrically (included with quadriceps in Fig. 2.9) to limit the speed at which the knee flexes. This eccentric contraction absorbs power (K3 in Fig. 2.7). At the ankle, the internal plantarflexor moment reduces rapidly during pre-swing as the magnitude of the ground reaction force declines, falling to zero as the foot leaves the ground at toe off (Fig. 2.6). The ankle power generation peak also declines to around zero during this period (Fig. 2.7).

Feet adjacent (Fig. 2.17)

1. General: Feet adjacent separates initial swing from mid-swing. It is the time when the swinging leg passes the stance phase leg and the two feet are side by side. The swing phase occupies about 40% of the gait cycle and the feet become adjacent around the center of this time; in the subject used for illustration, it occurred at 77% of the gait cycle. Alternative names for feet

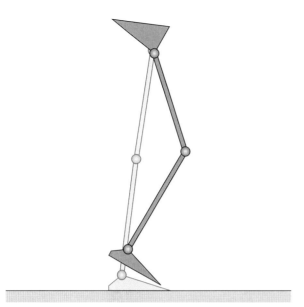

Fig. 2.17 Feet adjacent: position of right leg (gray) and left leg (blue).

adjacent are 'foot clearance' and 'mid-swing'; the latter term is now applied to a period of the gait cycle, rather than to a particular event. Initial swing is also known as 'lift off'.

2. Upper body: When the feet are adjacent, the trunk is at its highest position and is maximally displaced over the stance phase leg (left). The arms are level with each other, one (left) moving forward and one (right) moving back.

3. Hip: The hip starts to flex even prior to toe off and by the time the feet are adjacent, it is well flexed (20° in Fig. 2.5). This is achieved by a powerful contraction of iliopsoas (Fig. 2.9), aided by gravity.

4. Knee: The flexion of the knee during the swing phase results largely from the flexion of the hip. As described above (p. 76, toe off, section 6), the leg acts as a jointed pendulum and no muscular contraction is necessary around the knee (thus enabling above-knee amputees to achieve swing phase knee flexion in their prosthetic limb). The peak swing phase knee flexion angle is usually between 60° and 70°. It occurs before the feet are adjacent, by which time the knee has started to extend again. In fast walking, swing phase knee flexion is less than when walking at a natural speed, to shorten the swing phase. This is achieved by co-contraction of the rectus femoris and hamstrings (Gage, 2004, p. 58).

5. Ankle and foot: At the time the feet are adjacent, the ankle is moving from a plantarflexed attitude around toe off towards a neutral or dorsiflexed attitude in terminal swing. Most of the shortening of the swing phase leg required to achieve toe clearance comes from flexion of the knee, but the ankle also needs to move out of plantarflexion. This movement requires contraction of the anterior tibial muscles, although the force of contraction is much less than that required to control foot lowering following initial contact. The closest approach of the toes to the ground occurs around the time the feet are adjacent. In normal walking, the toes clear the ground by very little; Murray (1967) found a mean clearance of 14 mm with a range of 1–38 mm. The degree of foot supination reduces following toe off, but the foot remains slightly supinated until the following initial contact.

6. Moments and powers: As the hip moves into flexion, from opposite initial contact, through pre-swing and initial swing until the feet are adjacent, an internal flexor moment is present (Fig. 2.6). This is generated by gravity, rectus femoris and the adductors, with the addition of ligament elasticity at the beginning of the movement and iliopsoas contraction towards its end (Fig. 2.9). Hip flexion, in response to this moment, results in the highest peak of power generation at the hip (H3 in Fig. 2.7), the power being used to accelerate the swinging leg forward. The resulting kinetic energy is later transferred to the trunk, as the swinging leg is decelerated again at the end of the swing phase. Between toe off and feet adjacent, the knee continues to show a small internal extensor moment, as rectus femoris (part of quadriceps in Fig. 2.9) prevents the knee from flexing too rapidly in response to the external flexor moment transferred from the hip (see above). While the knee is still flexing, power absorption occurs (K3 in Fig. 2.7). Only very small moments and power exchanges are seen at the ankle, since only the weight of the foot is involved.

Tibia vertical (Fig. 2.18)

1. General: The division between the periods of mid-swing and terminal swing is marked by the tibia of the swinging leg becoming vertical, which occurred at 86% of the gait cycle in the subject used for illustration. Terminal swing is also known as 'reach'.

2. Upper body: When the tibia is vertical on the swing phase leg (right), the trunk has begun to lose vertical height and to move from its maximum displacement over the supporting (left) leg back towards the midline. The left arm is now in front of the right and the right side of the pelvis is a little in front of the left side (Fig. 2.18).

3. Hip: Tibia vertical marks approximately the time at which further hip flexion ceases, the subject used for illustration having a hip angle of about 27°

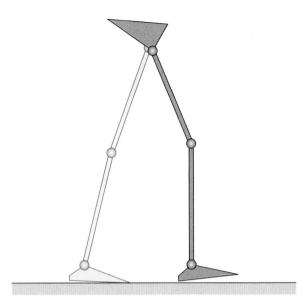

Fig. 2.18 Tibia vertical: position of right leg (gray) and left leg (blue).

of flexion from tibia vertical to the next initial contact (Fig. 2.5). The hamstrings contract increasingly strongly during terminal swing (Fig. 2.9) to limit the rate of knee extension, while maintaining the hip joint in this flexed position.

4. Knee: Tibia vertical occurs during a period of rapid knee extension, as the knee goes from the peak of swing phase flexion, prior to feet adjacent, to more or less full extension prior to the next initial contact (Fig. 2.5). This extension is largely passive, being the return swing of the lower (shank) segment of the double pendulum referred to above (p. 76, toe off, section 4). Eccentric contraction of the hamstrings prevents this motion from causing an abrupt hyperextension of the knee at the end of swing (Fig. 2.9).

5. Ankle and foot: Once toe clearance has occurred, generally before the tibia becomes vertical, the ankle attitude becomes less important: it may be anywhere between a few degrees of plantarflexion and a few degrees of dorsiflexion, prior to the next initial contact (Fig. 2.5). Tibialis anterior continues to contract, to hold the ankle in position, but its activity usually increases prior to initial contact, in anticipation of the greater contraction forces which will be needed during the loading response (Fig. 2.9).

6. Moments and powers: At the hip, by the time of tibia vertical, an increasing internal extensor moment is seen (Fig. 2.6), largely generated by contraction of the hamstrings, although gluteus maximus also begins to contract prior to the next initial contact (Fig. 2.9). This moment probably permits the transfer of momentum from the swinging leg to the trunk, recovering some of the kinetic energy imparted to the leg in initial swing (H3 in Fig. 2.7). Since the hip angle is essentially static during terminal swing, very little power exchange occurs at the joint itself. The knee demonstrates an increasing internal flexor moment (Fig. 2.6), which is generated by eccentric contraction of the hamstrings (Fig. 2.9), with power absorption (K4 in Fig. 2.7). This occurs in response to an external extensor moment, generated by the inertia of the swinging shank, which would hyperextend the knee if it were not checked. The ankle moment remains negligible (Fig. 2.6), with very little power exchange (Fig. 2.7).

Terminal foot contact (Fig. 2.10)

The gait cycle ends at the next initial contact of the same foot (in this case, the right foot). Because it is confusing to refer to the *end* of the cycle as '*initial contact*', it is sometimes known as 'terminal foot contact'.

GROUND REACTION FORCES

The *force platform* (or forceplate) is an instrument commonly used in gait analysis. It gives the total force applied by the foot to the ground, although it does not show the distribution of different parts of this force (e.g. heel and forefoot) on the walking surface. Some force platforms give only one component of the force (usually vertical), but most give a full three-dimensional description of the ground reaction force vector. The electrical output signals may be processed to produce three components of force (vertical, lateral and fore–aft), the two coordinates of the center of pressure and the moments about the vertical axis. The *center of pressure* is the point on the ground through which a single resultant force appears to act, although in reality the total force is made up of innumerable small force vectors, spread out across a finite area on the surface of the platform.

Since the ground reaction force is a three-dimensional vector, it would be preferable to display it as such for the purposes of interpretation. Unfortunately, this is seldom practical. The most common form of display is that shown in Fig. 2.19, where the three components of force are plotted against time for the walk shown in the previous figures. The sign convention used in Fig. 2.19 is the same as that used by Winter (1991), where the ground reaction force is positive upwards, forwards and to the right. Regrettably there is no general agreement on sign conventions.

The lateral component of force is generally very small; for most of the stance phase of the right foot, the ground reaction force accelerates the center of gravity towards the left side of the body, and during the stance phase of the

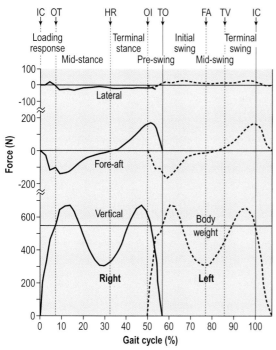

Fig. 2.19 Lateral, fore–aft and vertical components of the ground reaction force, in newtons, for right foot (solid line) and left foot (dashed line). Abbreviations as in Fig. 2.5. See text for sign conventions.

left foot, the acceleration is towards the right side of the body. The fore–aft (or anteroposterior) trace from the right foot shows 'braking' during the first half of the stance phase and 'propulsion' during the second half. The left foot shows the same pattern, but with the direction of the lateral force reversed. The vertical force shows a characteristic double hump, which results from an upward acceleration of the center of gravity during early stance, a reduction in downward force as the body 'flies' over the leg in mid-stance and a second peak due to deceleration, as the downward motion is checked in late stance.

Plots of this type are difficult to interpret and encourage consideration of the force vector as separate components, rather than as a three-dimensional whole. The 'butterfly diagram' shown in Fig. 2.8 is an improvement on this, since it combines two of the force components (vertical and fore–aft) with the center of pressure in the fore–aft direction. It also preserves information on timing, since the lines representing the force vector are at regular intervals (10 ms in this case). Butterfly diagrams for the frontal and transverse planes are more difficult to interpret and are seldom if ever used.

The other type of information commonly derived from the force platform is the position of the center of pressure of the two feet on the ground, as shown in Fig. 2.20, again for the same walk. This may be used to identify abnormal patterns of foot contact, including an abnormal toe out or toe in angle. The

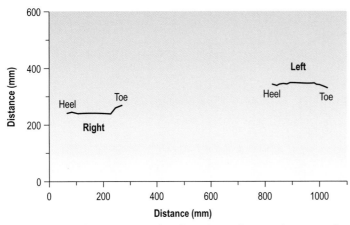

Fig. 2.20 View of the walking surface from above, showing the center of pressure beneath the two feet, with the right heel contacting first and the subject walking towards the right of the diagram.

step length and walking base can also be measured from this type of display, providing there is an identifiable initial contact.

Should the pattern of foot contact be of particular interest, it is preferable to combine the data on the center of pressure with an outline of the foot, obtained by some other means (such as chalk on the floor). This type of display, with the addition of a sagittal plane representation of the ground reaction force vector, is shown in Fig. 2.21 for a normal male subject wearing shoes. The trace shows initial contact at the back of the heel on the lateral side, with progression of the center of force along the middle of the foot to the metatarsal heads, where it moves medially, ending at the hallux. The spacing of the vectors shows how long the center of pressure spends in any one area. It is worth noting that there is a cluster of vectors just in front of the edge of the heel, where the shoe is not in contact with the ground, again pointing out the fact that the center of pressure is merely the average of a number of forces acting beneath the foot.

There is considerable variation between individuals as to how much force is applied to the ground at initial contact, some people 'gliding' the foot onto the ground and others 'digging' it in. Figure 2.22 shows the vertical component of the ground reaction force from a fast walk, in hard-heeled shoes, by an individual with a marked heelstrike. The data were recorded at 1000 Hz from a Bertec force platform, which has a particularly high-frequency response. It has been suggested that transient forces in the joints, resulting from the heelstrike, may cause degenerative arthritis (Radin, 1987). The heelstrike transient represents the transfer of momentum from the moving leg to the ground. It is a fairly short event, typically lasting 10–20 ms, and can only be observed using measuring equipment with a fast enough response time. The present author has published a review article on the heelstrike transient and related topics (Whittle, 1999).

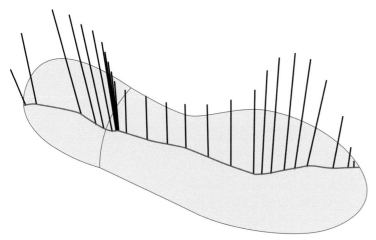

Fig. 2.21 Foot outline, center of pressure and sagittal plane representation of ground reaction force vector; right foot of a normal male subject walking in shoes.

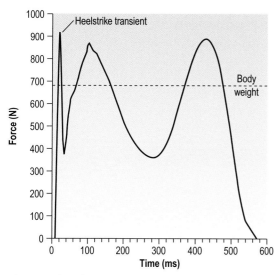

Fig. 2.22 Plot of vertical ground reaction force against time, showing the heelstrike transient in a particularly 'vigorous' walker wearing hard-heeled shoes. Unfiltered data from Bertec force platform, sampled at 1000 Hz.

Moments about the vertical axis are seldom reported. In comparing these moments between normal children with children with clubfeet, Sawatzky *et al.* (1994) were surprised to find only small, and not statistically significant, differences. However, as will be explained in Chapter 4, these moments largely result from the acceleration and deceleration of the swing phase leg and only minor changes could be expected to be introduced by the foot on the ground.

SUPPORT MOMENT

Winter (1980) coined the term 'support moment' to describe the sum of the sagittal plane moments about the hip, knee and ankle joints:

$$M_S = M_H + M_K + M_A \qquad \text{(Winter)}$$

where M_S, M_H, M_K and M_A are the support, hip, knee and ankle moments, respectively.

Winter noted that the support moment was far less variable than its individual components, suggesting that a decreased moment about one joint could be compensated for by an increased moment about one or both of the other joints. However, it was difficult to interpret this in biomechanical terms, since the sign convention was based on flexion and extension, rather than on clockwise and counterclockwise moments, which caused the direction of the knee moment to be opposite to that of the hip and ankle moments. Hof (2000) published a justification for the support moment and suggested that it is responsible for preventing collapse of the knee. Based on his analysis, he suggested the following revised formula for its calculation:

$$M_S = \tfrac{1}{2}M_H + M_K + \tfrac{1}{2}M_A \qquad \text{(Hof)}$$

Figure 2.23 illustrates the support moment calculated from the sagittal plane hip, knee and ankle internal moments from the normal subject used for illustration throughout this chapter, using the formula suggested by Hof (2000).

Anderson & Pandy (2003) suggested that a better alternative to the support moment would be the sum of the vertical components of force from individual muscles during walking.

ENERGY CONSUMPTION

It is relatively easy to measure the energy consumption of a vehicle, but much more difficult to make equivalent measurements of human walking, for two reasons. Firstly, there is a clear relationship between the fuel level in the tank of a vehicle and how much energy has been used, whereas knowing how much food a person has eaten gives no information on the energy consumed in a particular activity. Secondly, a vehicle which is switched off uses no energy, whereas people use metabolic energy all the time, whether they are walking or not.

The first problem, that of measuring the 'fuel consumption', can be solved by measuring not the fuel consumed but the oxygen which is used to oxidize

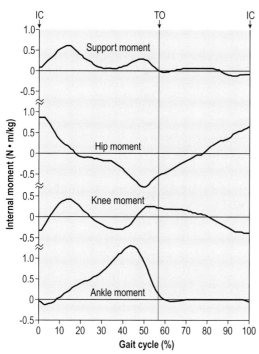

Fig. 2.23 Support moment, calculated using the formula of Hof (2000), from the sagittal plane internal joint moments of right hip, knee and ankle. Abbreviations and sign conventions as in Fig. 2.6.

it. Measurements of oxygen uptake, while not particularly pleasant for the subject (who has to wear a face mask or mouthpiece), are nonetheless perfectly practical and are used routinely to measure the metabolic cost of different activities.

The second problem, the lack of a suitable baseline for energy consumption measurements in humans, is not easy to solve and requires a different way of thinking about the topic. The energy used by a person who is walking can be divided into three parts.

1. The muscles used for walking consume energy, as they accelerate and decelerate the trunk and the limb segments in different directions.
2. There is an 'overhead' involved in walking, in that the expenditure of energy by the muscles involves increased activity by the heart and the muscles used in breathing, which themselves use energy. Energy is also expended in maintaining the upright posture.
3. The 'basal metabolism' is the irreducible minimum energy a person will consume if they are totally at rest.

The relationship between metabolic energy and physical energy is very complicated. As explained in Chapter 1 (p. 43), if a muscle undergoes an isometric contraction, it still uses energy, although its length does not change and the physical work it does is zero. In an eccentric contraction, when it lengthens under tension, it uses up metabolic energy, when in physical terms one would expect it to gain energy, rather than to lose it.

In the past it has been usual to estimate the mechanical efficiency of walking by looking at the difference in oxygen consumption between the 'basal' state and walking at a given speed. This approach neglects the various overheads, however, and makes slow walking appear to be extremely inefficient. Inman *et al.* (1981) and Rose & Gamble (1994) suggested that it is more realistic to use standing or very slow walking as the baseline for measurements of faster walking. Despite these uncertainties, a figure of 25% is often quoted for the efficiency of the conversion of metabolic energy into mechanical energy in a wide range of activities, including walking. A comprehensive review of the energy expenditure of normal and pathological gait was given by Waters & Mulroy (1999).

The energy requirements of walking can be expressed in two ways: the energy used per unit time and the energy used per unit distance. Since energy expenditure is usually inferred from the oxygen used, these are generally known as 'oxygen consumption' and 'oxygen cost', respectively.

Energy consumption per unit time (oxygen consumption)

Inman *et al.* (1981) and Rose & Gamble (1994) quoted an equation, based on a number of studies, for the relationship between the walking speed and the energy consumption per unit time. The energy consumption included both the basal metabolism and the 'overheads'. They showed, not surprisingly, that energy consumption per unit time is less for slow walking than for fast walking. Translating their equation into SI units, it becomes:

$$E_w = 2.23 + 1.26\ v^2$$

where E_w is the energy consumption in watts per kilogram body mass and v is the speed in m/s.

As an example of the application of this equation, a 70 kg person walking at 1.4 m/s, which is a typical speed for adults, would consume energy at a rate of 330 w. The term v^2 in the equation shows that energy consumption increases as the square of the walking speed.

Energy consumption per unit distance (oxygen cost)

The energy consumption per meter walked, also known as 'energy cost', has a less straightforward relationship with walking speed, as both very slow and very fast walking speeds use more energy per meter than walking at intermediate speeds. The equation which describes this relationship, again converted into SI units, is:

$$E_m = 2.23/v + 1.26\,v$$

where E_m is the energy consumption in joules per meter per kilogram body mass and v is the speed in m/s. The energy cost of walking is higher in children and decreases steadily with age up to adulthood.

The minimum energy usage is predicted by this equation at a speed of 1.33 m/s. A 70 kg person walking at this speed would use 235 joules per meter, or 235 kJ per kilometer. A typical 'candy' bar contains around 1000 kJ and would thus supply enough energy to walk 4.26 km, or more than two and a half miles!

The equations quoted above merely give average values for adults, which may be modified by age, sex, walking surface, footwear and so on. Pathological gait is frequently associated with an energy consumption considerably above these 'average' values, due to some combination of abnormal movements, muscle spasticity and co-contraction of antagonistic muscles. To provide a baseline for studies of pathological gait, Waters *et al.* (1988) made a detailed study of the energy consumption of a total of 260 normal children and adults of both sexes, walking at a variety of speeds.

OPTIMIZATION OF ENERGY USAGE

If people were fitted with wheels, very little energy would be needed for locomotion on a level surface and some of the energy expended in going uphill would be recovered when coming down again. For this reason, both wheelchairs and bicycles are remarkably efficient forms of transport, although obviously much less versatile than a pair of legs. During walking, each leg in turn has to be started and stopped and the center of gravity of the body rises and falls and moves from side to side, all of which use energy. Despite this, walking is not as inefficient as it might be, due to two forms of optimization: those involving transfers of energy and those which minimize the displacement of the center of gravity.

Energy transfers

Two types of energy transfer occur during walking: an exchange between potential and kinetic energy and the transfer of energy between one limb segment and another. The most obvious exchange between potential and kinetic energy is in the movement of the trunk. During the double support phase, the trunk is at its lowest vertical position, with its highest forward speed. During the first half of the single support phase, the trunk is lifted up by the supporting leg, converting some of its kinetic energy into potential energy, as its speed reduces. During the latter part of the single support phase, the trunk drops down again in front of the supporting leg and reduces its height while picking up speed again. These exchanges between potential and kinetic energy are the same as in a child's swing, in which the potential energy at the highest point in its travel is converted into kinetic energy as it swings downwards, then back into potential energy again as it swings up the other side.

As well as the vertical motion of the trunk, there are other exchanges between potential and kinetic energy in walking. The twisting of the shoulder girdle and pelvis in opposite directions stores potential energy as tension in the elastic structures, which is converted to kinetic energy as the trunk untwists and then back to potential energy again as the trunk twists the other way.

Winter *et al.* (1976) studied the energy levels of the limb segments and of the quaintly named HAT (Head, Arms and Trunk). These authors criticized some earlier studies, which had included the kinetic energy of linear motion but neglected the kinetic energy due to rotation, which is responsible for about 10% of the total energy of the shank. Winter *et al.* studied only the sagittal plane, regarding energy exchanges in the other planes as negligible. They confirmed the exchange between potential and kinetic energy, described above, and estimated that roughly half of the energy of the HAT segment was conserved in this way. The thigh conserved about a third of its energy by exchanges of this sort and the shank virtually none. They also noted that the changes in total body energy were less than the changes in energy of the individual segments, indicating a transfer of energy from one segment to another. In one subject, during a single gait cycle, the energy changes were: shank 16 J, thigh 6 J and HAT 10 J, making a total of 32 J. However, the total body energy change was only 22 J, indicating a saving of 10 J by intersegment transfers.

Siegel *et al.* (2004) performed a detailed analysis on the relationship between lower limb joint moments and mechanical energy during gait.

The six determinants of gait

The six optimizations used to minimize the excursions of the center of gravity were called the 'determinants of gait' by Saunders *et al.* (1953), in a classic paper the main points of which were reiterated, with slight changes, by Inman *et al.* (1981) and Rose & Gamble (1994). A brief description is given below, but one of these sources should be consulted for a detailed and well-illustrated account. The fourth and fifth determinants were combined in the original descriptions but for the purposes of clarity, the present author has separated them and made other minor changes.

For more than 40 years after their first publication, the determinants of gait were generally accepted and have been redescribed in numerous publications, including previous editions of the present book. However, it has more recently been suggested, in a series of publications (e.g. Della Croce *et al.*, 2001; Gard & Childress, 1997), that although these motions certainly occur, some of them may play little or no part in reducing energy expenditure. Kerrigan (2003) suggested that only the fifth determinant of gait (foot mechanism) significantly reduces the vertical excursions of the center of mass. Baker *et al.* (2004) rejected the notion that energy is conserved by restricting the vertical movements of the center of gravity and proposed instead that energy is mainly conserved by a backwards-and-forwards exchange between potential energy and kinetic energy, as described above. However, having provided these warnings, I will nonetheless reiterate the original descriptions by Saunders *et al.* (1953)!

The six 'determinants of gait' are as follows.

1. Pelvic rotation: If the knee is kept straight, a movement of the hip from a flexed position to an extended one, such as occurs in the stance phase of gait, will result in the hip joint moving forwards, but also in its rising and then falling again. The amount of forward movement and the amount of rising and falling both depend on the total angle through which the hip joint moves from flexion to extension (Fig. 2.24, left). Since the forward movement is equal to

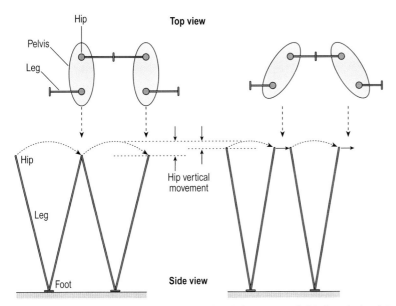

Fig 2.24 First determinant of gait: if the pelvis did not rotate (left), the whole of the stride length would come from hip flexion and extension. Pelvic rotation about a vertical axis (right) reduces the angle of hip flexion and extension, which in turn reduces the vertical movement of the hip.

the stride length, it follows that the greater the stride length, the greater will be the angles of flexion and extension of the hip, and the more the hip will move vertically between its highest and lowest positions. The first 'determinant of gait' is the way in which the pelvis twists about a vertical axis during the gait cycle, bringing each hip joint forwards as that hip flexes and backwards as it extends. This means that for a given stride length, the hip joint itself moves forward through a smaller distance than the foot, so that less flexion and extension of the hip is required. A proportion of the stride length thus comes from the forward-and-backward movement of the hip joint. The reduction in the range of hip flexion and extension leads to a reduction in the vertical movement of the hip (Fig. 2.24, right).

2. Pelvic obliquity: As described above, flexion and extension of the hip are accompanied by a rise and fall in the height of the hip joint. If the pelvis were to keep level, the trunk would follow this up-and-down movement. However, the second 'determinant of gait' is the way in which the pelvis tips about an anteroposterior axis, raising first one side and then the other, so that when the hip of the stance phase leg is at its highest point, the pelvis slopes downwards, so that the hip of the swing phase leg is lower than that of the stance phase leg. Since the height of the trunk does not depend on the height of either hip joint alone but on the average of the two of them, this pelvic obliquity reduces the total vertical excursion of the trunk (Fig. 2.25). However, it can only be achieved if the swing phase leg can be shortened sufficiently to clear the ground (normally by both flexing the knee and dorsiflexing the ankle), when the height of its hip joint is reduced.

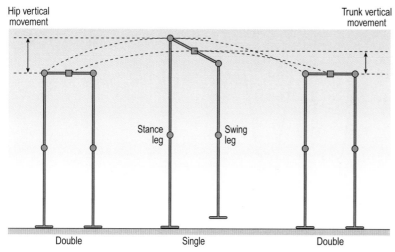

Fig. 2.25 Second determinant of gait: the vertical movement of the trunk is less than that of the hip, due to pelvic tilt about an anteroposterior axis.

3. Knee flexion in stance phase: The third, fourth and fifth determinants of gait (Fig. 2.26) are all concerned with adjusting the effective length of the leg, by lengthening it at the beginning and end of the stance phase and shortening it in the middle, to keep the hip height as constant as possible. The third 'determinant' is the stance phase flexion of the knee. As the femur passes from flexion of the hip into extension, if the leg remained straight, the hip joint would rise and then fall, as described above. However, flexion of the knee shortens the leg in the middle of this movement, reducing the height of the apex of the curve.

4. Ankle mechanism: Complementary to the way in which the apex of the curve is lowered by shortening the leg in the middle of the movement from hip flexion to extension, the beginning of the curve is elevated by lengthening the leg at the start of the stance phase – initial contact. This is achieved by the fourth 'determinant of gait' – the ankle mechanism. Because the heel sticks out behind the ankle joint, it effectively lengthens the leg during the loading response (Fig. 2.26).

5. Foot mechanism: In the same way that the heel lengthens the leg at the start of the stance phase, the forefoot lengthens it at the end of stance, in the fifth 'determinant' – the terminal rocker (Fig. 2.26). From the time of heel rise, the effective length of the lower leg increases as the ankle moves from dorsiflexion into plantarflexion.

6. Lateral displacement of body: The first five determinants of gait are all concerned with reducing the vertical excursions of the center of gravity. The sixth is concerned with side-to-side movement. If the feet were as far apart as the hips, the body would need to tip from side to side to maintain balance

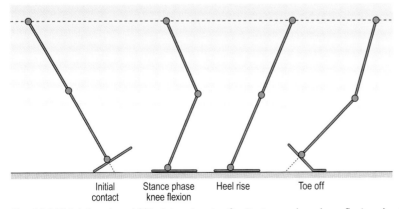

Initial contact   Stance phase knee flexion   Heel rise   Toe off

Fig. 2.26 Third, fourth and fifth determinants of gait: stance phase knee flexion shortens the leg in mid-stance (third determinant); backward projection of the heel at initial contact lengthens the leg (fourth determinant); so does forward projection of the forefoot during pre-swing (fifth determinant).

during walking (Fig. 2.27a). By keeping the walking base narrow, little lateral movement is needed to preserve balance (Fig. 2.27b). The reduction in lateral acceleration and deceleration leads to a reduction in the use of muscular energy. The main adaptation which allows the walking base to be narrow is a slight valgus angulation of the knee, which permits the tibia to be vertical while the femur inclines inwards, from a slightly adducted hip.

It should be obvious that although the six determinants of gait have been described separately, they are all integrated together during each gait cycle. The combined effect is a much smoother trajectory for the center of gravity and (according to the original description) a much lower energy expenditure. According to Perry (1992), the determinants of gait reduce the vertical excursions of the trunk by about 50% and the horizontal excursions by about 40%.

STARTING AND STOPPING

To this point, only steady-state continuous walking has been considered. In order to achieve that state, the individual has to start off, and when they reach

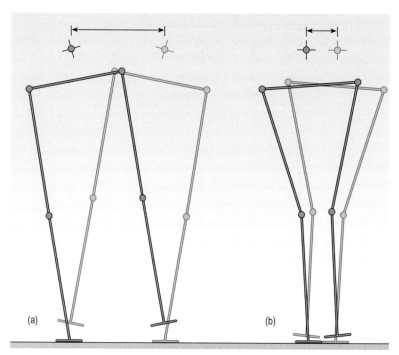

Fig. 2.27 Sixth determinant of gait: if the feet are placed on the ground far apart (a), large side-to-side movements of the center of gravity would be necessary to maintain balance; having them closer together (b) reduces the size of these movements.

their destination, they have to stop. Winter (1995), in a review of balance and posture control, gave a good description of gait initiation and gait termination.

In gait initiation, from standing on both feet, the body weight is shifted to one foot, thus permitting the other foot to be lifted off the ground and moved forward. As an example, suppose the left foot was going to move forwards first (swing limb), while the body weight is supported by the right foot (stance limb). The shifting of weight over the right foot is achieved by a brief initial push, backwards and to the left, by the left foot. This (following Newton's second law) moves the center of gravity of the body forwards and to the right. Once the center of gravity is over the right foot, it is safe to lift the left foot off the ground and move it forward. At the same time, the trunk has started to move forward. The left foot lands on the ground in front of the subject, with a step that is almost exactly the same as in steady-state gait. Body weight is transferred to the left leg, the right foot leaves the ground with a normal toe off, and the subject is walking. By the time the left foot has contacted the ground, the trunk is moving forward at around 85% of the final walking speed and only one or two more steps are needed before the steady-state speed and pattern are achieved. Probably the slowest adjustment is that of side-to-side balance, which may need several steps to stabilize.

A pathology which causes particular problems for the initiation of gait is parkinsonism; gait initiation in this condition was reviewed by Halliday *et al.* (1998).

Less research has been done on gait termination, although it appears to present a greater challenge to the neural control system. Gait termination involves a stance phase on one side, which is not followed by a swing phase, and a shortened swing phase on the other, the moving foot being placed beside the stationary one. If the left foot is the swinging one, the forces to terminate gait are provided by the right foot, which directs the ground reaction force forward and to the right, thus applying a backwards and leftwards force to the body center of gravity, arresting its forward motion and bringing it to the midpoint between the feet. The left foot is then planted on the ground beside the right one and the walk has terminated.

OTHER VARIETIES OF GAIT

As well as normal walking, humans walk backwards, skip, run, ascend and descend slopes and stairs, step over obstacles and carry loads in their hands, on their backs or on their heads. Running has an extensive literature of its own, since it is such an important part of sports medicine. The other types of locomotion have all been studied to a greater or lesser extent, particularly because patients with abnormal neuromuscular systems frequently have greater problems with some of these other activities than they do with normal walking. However, such considerations are beyond the scope of the present introductory text.

GAIT IN THE YOUNG

Although a number of studies have been made of the development of gait in children, that by Sutherland *et al.* (1988) is one of the most detailed. The main ways in which the gait of small children differs from that of adults are as follows:

1. The walking base is wider
2. The stride length and speed are lower and the cycle time shorter (higher cadence)
3. Small children have no heelstrike, initial contact being made by the flat foot
4. There is very little stance phase knee flexion
5. The whole leg is externally rotated during the swing phase
6. There is an absence of reciprocal arm swinging.

These differences in gait mature at different rates. The characteristics numbered (3), (4) and (5) in the above list have changed to the adult pattern by the age of 2, and (1) and (6) by the age of 4. The cycle time, stride length and speed continue to change with growth, reaching normal adult values around the age of 15.

Most children commence walking within 3 months of their first birthday. Prior to this, even tiny babies will make reciprocal stepping motions, if they are moved slowly forwards while held in the standing position with their feet on the ground. However, this is not true walking, as there is little attempt to take any weight on the legs.

Figure 2.28, which is based on data from Sutherland *et al.* (1988), shows the average sagittal plane motion at the hip, knee and ankle joints in 49 children between 11 and 13 months. It should be compared with Fig. 2.5, which shows the same parameters for a normal adult female. Sutherland *et al.* only gave the timing of initial contact and toe off on the two sides and used a different definition of hip angle; the data in Fig. 2.28 have been adjusted into extension by 15° to make them comparable with the other figures in this book.

The pattern of hip flexion and extension differs from that in adults in that the degree of extension is reduced and the hip does not remain flexed for so long at the end of the swing phase.

The knee never fully extends, but this is seen at all ages in Sutherland's data and may reflect the method of measurement. There is some stance phase knee flexion in infants, but it is both smaller in magnitude and earlier than in adults. The flexion of the knee in the swing phase is also somewhat reduced at

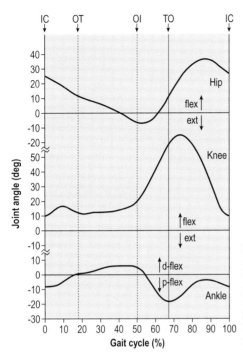

IC OT OI TO IC

Joint angle (deg)

Gait cycle (%)

Hip
flex
ext
Knee
flex
ext
d-flex
p-flex
Ankle

Fig. 2.28 Sagittal plane hip, knee and ankle angles in 1-year-old children. The hip angle has been moved into extension by 15° to allow for a difference in measurement methods. Sign conventions and abbreviations as in Fig. 2.5 (based on data from Sutherland *et al.*, 1988).

the age of 1 (and most adults have more swing phase flexion than is seen in Fig. 2.5).

Initial contact in small children is by the whole foot, heelstrike being replaced by foot flat. The ankle is plantarflexed at initial contact and remains so into the early stance phase, in contrast to the adult pattern, in which the ankle is approximately neutral at initial contact but moves rapidly into plantarflexion. The pattern of dorsiflexion followed by plantarflexion through the remainder of the stance phase is essentially the same at all ages.

Since children are smaller than adults, it is not surprising that they walk with a shorter stride length and at a slower speed. Sutherland *et al.* (1988) showed that stride length is closely related to height and that the ratio of stride length to stature is similar to that found in adults. The change in stride length with age mirrors the change in height, showing a rapid increase up to age 4 and a slower increase thereafter. Todd *et al.* (1989) detailed the relationships between the height of children and their general gait parameters. Small children walk with a short cycle time (rapid cadence), the mean at the age of one being about 0.70 s (171 steps/min). Cycle time increases with age but is still around 0.85 s (141 steps/min) at age 7, which is well below the typical adult values of 1.06 s (113 steps/min) for men and 1.02 s (118 steps/min) for women. The shorter cycle time partly compensates for the short stride length and the speed ranged from 0.64 m/s at age 1 to 1.14 m/s at age 7, compared with the typical adult values of 1.46 m/s for males and 1.3 m/s for females. Sutherland did not report on the gait of children beyond the age of 7 and did not distinguish between the results from boys and girls. Appendix 1 gives the normal ranges for the general gait parameters in children, derived in part from Sutherland's data. However, values based on age alone may be misleading; stride length depends on both height and walking speed, both of which may be lower in children with a disability than in normal children of the same age.

As can be seen in Fig. 2.28, the swing phase occupies a smaller proportion of the gait cycle in very small children than in adults, thus minimizing the time spent in the less stable condition of single legged stance. The relative duration of the swing phase increases with age, reaching the adult proportion around the age of 4 years. There is symmetry between the two sides at all ages. Sutherland *et al.* (1988) related the width of the walking base to the width of the body at the top of the pelvis, using the somewhat confusing 'pelvic-span/ankle-spread' ratio. Changing the measurement units for the sake of clarity, the walking base is about 70% of the pelvic width at the age of 1 year, falling to about 45% by the age of 3^1/$_2$, at which level it remains until the age of 7. An average value for adults is not readily available but it is probably less than 30%.

At the very youngest ages, the EMG patterns showed that there is a tendency to activate most muscles for a higher proportion of the gait cycle than in adults. With the exception of the triceps surae, adult patterns are established for most muscles by the age of 2. Sutherland *et al.* (1988) found that children could be divided into two groups depending on whether the triceps surae was activated in a prolonged (infant) pattern or the normal (adult) pattern. Below the age of 2, over 60% of the children showed the infant pattern; the proportion dropped to below 30% by the age of 7. The authors speculated that this might relate to delayed myelination of the sensory branches of the peripheral nerves.

An excellent review of the main changes in gait which occur during childhood was given by Sutherland (1997). The gait of very small children (under the age of 2) was examined in detail by Grimshaw *et al.* (1998). The joint moments and powers of this same group were studied by Hallemans *et al.* (2005).

GAIT IN THE ELDERLY

A number of investigations have been made of the changes in gait which occur with advancing age, especially by Murray *et al.* (1969), who studied the gait of men up to the age of 87. The description which follows is confined to the effects of age on free-speed walking, although Murray *et al.* also examined fast walking. A companion paper (Murray *et al.*, 1970) studied the gait of women up to age 70. It did not provide as much information on the effects of age, but generally confirmed the observations made on males.

The gait of the elderly is subject to two influences: the effects of age itself and the effects of pathological conditions, such as osteoarthritis and parkinsonism, which become more common with advancing age. Providing patients with pathological conditions are carefully excluded, the gait of the elderly appears to be simply a 'slowed down' version of the gait of younger adults. Murray *et al.* (1969) were careful to point out that 'the walking performance of older men did not resemble a pathological gait'.

Typically, the onset of age-related changes in gait takes place in the decade from 60 to 70 years of age. There is a decreased stride length, a variable but generally increased cycle time (decreased cadence) and an increase in the walking base. Many other changes can also be observed, such as a relative increase in the duration of the stance phase as a percentage of the gait cycle, but most of them are secondary to the changes in stride length, cycle time and walking base. The speed (stride length divided by cycle time) is almost always reduced in elderly people. Appendix 1 gives normal ranges for the general gait parameters up to the age of 80.

Some of the differences between the gait of the young and the elderly are apparent in Fig. 2.29, which is taken from Murray *et al.* (1969). These authors suggested that the purpose of gait changes in the elderly is to improve the security of walking. Both decreasing the stride length and increasing the walking base make it easier to maintain balance while walking. Increasing the cycle time (reducing the cadence) leads to a reduction in the percentage of the gait cycle for which there is only single limb support, since the increase in cycle length is largely achieved by lengthening the stance phase and hence the double support time.

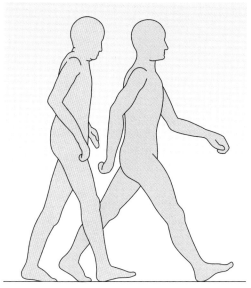

Fig. 2.29 Body position at right initial contact in older men (left) and younger men (right) (Murray *et al.*, 1969).

Changes in the angular excursions of the joints in the elderly include a reduction in the total range of hip flexion and extension, a reduction in swing phase knee flexion and reduced ankle plantarflexion during the push off. However, all of these depend on both cycle time and stride length and are probably within normal limits if these factors are taken into account. Nigg *et al.* (1994) confirmed these observations in a detailed study on three-dimensional joint ranges of motion in walking, in male and female subjects from 20 to 79 years of age.

The vertical movement of the head is reduced and its lateral movement increased, probably secondary to the changes in stride length and walking base, respectively.

The trajectory of the toe over the ground is modified in old age, giving an improved ground clearance during the first half of the swing phase. This is probably another mechanism for improving security. The heel rises less during pre-swing and the foot attitude is closer to the horizontal at initial contact, both of these changes being related to the reduction in stride length. There is also an increase in the angle of toe out in elderly people and changes in the posture and movements of the arms, the elbows being more flexed and the shoulders more extended. The reasons for these differences are not known.

The dividing line between normal and abnormal may be difficult to define in elderly people. A condition known as 'idiopathic gait disorder of the elderly' has been described, which is essentially an exaggeration of the gait changes which normally occur with age and is characterized by a cautious attitude to walking, with a prolonged cycle time (low cadence), a short stride length and an increased step-to-step variability. A comprehensive review of the changes in gait with advancing age was given by Prince *et al.* (1997).

References and suggestions for further reading

Anderson FC, Pandy MG. (2003) Individual muscle contributions to support in normal walking. *Gait and Posture* **17**: 159–169.

Baker R, Kirkwood C, Pandy M. (2004) Minimizing the vertical excursion of the center of mass is not the primary aim of walking. Eighth International Symposium on the 3-D Analysis of Human Movement, Tampa, Florida, USA, March 31–April 2, pp. 101–104.

Blanc Y, Balmer C, Landis T, Vingerhoets F. (1999) Temporal parameters and patterns of foot roll over during walking: normative data for healthy adults. *Gait and Posture* **10**: 97–108.

Bresler B, Frankel JP. (1950) The forces and moments in the leg during level walking. *American Society of Mechanical Engineers Transactions* **72**: 27–36.

Buczek FL, Sanders JO, Concha MC *et al.* (2003) Inadequacy of an inverted pendulum model of human gait. Gait and Clinical Movement Analysis Society, Eighth Annual Meeting, Wilmington, Delaware, USA, pp. 185–186.

Burnfield JM, Tsai Y-J, Powers CM. (2005) Comparison of utilized coefficient of friction during different walking tasks in persons with and without a disability. *Gait and Posture* **22**: 82–88.

Cavagna GA, Margaria R. (1966) Mechanics of walking. *Journal of Applied Physiology* **21**: 271–278.

Cham R, Redfern MS. (2002) Changes in gait when anticipating slippery floors. *Gait and Posture* **15**: 159–171.

Della Croce U, Riley PO, Lelas JL *et al.* (2001) A refined view of the determinants of gait. *Gait and Posture* **14**: 79–84.

Gage JR (ed). (2004) *The Treatment of Gait Problems in Cerebral Palsy.* London: MacKeith Press.

Gard SA, Childress DS. (1997) The effect of pelvic list on the vertical displacement of the trunk during normal walking. *Gait and Posture* **5**: 233–238.

Garrison FH. (1929) *An Introduction to the History of Medicine.* Philadelphia, PA: W.B. Saunders Co.

Grimshaw PN, Marques-Bruna P, Salo A *et al.* (1998) The 3-dimensional kinematics of the walking gait cycle of children aged between 10 and 24 months: cross sectional and repeated measures. *Gait and Posture* **7**: 7–15.

Hallemans A, De Clercq D, Otten B *et al.* (2005) 3D joint dynamics of walking in toddlers. A cross-sectional study spanning the first rapid development phase of walking. *Gait and Posture* **22**: 107–118.

Halliday SE, Winter DA, Frank JS *et al.* (1998) The initiation of gait in young, elderly and Parkinson's disease subjects. *Gait and Posture* **8**: 8–14.

Hof AL. (2000) On the interpretation of the support moment. *Gait and Posture* **12**: 196–199.

Inman VT, Ralston HJ, Todd F. (1981) *Human Walking.* Baltimore, MD: Williams and Wilkins.

Kerrigan CD. (2003) Discoveries from quantitative gait analysis. *Gait and Posture* **18** (Suppl. 1): S13.

Lamoth CJC, Beek PJ, Meijer OG. (2002) Pelvis–thorax coordination in the transverse plane during gait. *Gait and Posture* **16**: 101–114.

Macellari V, Giacomozzi C, Saggini R. (1999) Spatial–temporal parameters of gait: reference data and a statistical method for normality assessment. *Gait and Posture* **10**: 171–181.

Mueller MJ, Sinacore DR, Hoogstrate S *et al.* (1994) Hip and ankle walking strategies: effect on peak plantar pressures and implications for neuropathic ulceration. *Archives of Physical Medicine and Rehabilitation* **75**: 1196–1200.

Murray MP. (1967) Gait as a total pattern of movement. *American Journal of Physical Medicine* **46**: 290–333.

Murray MP, Kory RC, Clarkson BH. (1969) Walking patterns in healthy old men. *Journal of Gerontology* **24**: 169–178.

Murray MP, Kory RC, Sepic SB. (1970) Walking patterns of normal women. *Archives of Physical Medicine and Rehabilitation* **51**: 637–650.

Nene A, Mayagoitia R, Veltink P. (1999) Assessment of rectus femoris function during initial swing phase. *Gait and Posture* **9**: 1–9.

Nigg BM, Fisher V, Ronsky JL. (1994) Gait characteristics as a function of age and gender. *Gait and Posture* **2**: 213–220.

Oeffinger D, Brauch B, Cranfill S *et al.* (1999) Comparison of gait with and without shoes in children. *Gait and Posture* **9**: 95–100.

Paul JP. (1965) Bio-engineering studies of the forces transmitted by joints. (II) Engineering analysis. In: Kenedi JP (ed.) *Biomechanics and Related Bioengineering Topics.* Oxford: Pergamon, pp. 369–380.

Paul JP. (1966) Forces transmitted by joints in the human body. *Proceedings of the Institute of Mechanical Engineers* **181**: 8–15.

Pedotti A. (1977) Simple equipment used in clinical practice for the evaluation of locomotion. *IEEE Transactions on Biomedical Engineering* **BME-24**: 456–461.

Perry J. (1974) Kinesiology of lower extremity bracing. *Clinical Orthopaedics and Related Research* **102**: 18–31.

Perry J. (1992) *Gait Analysis: Normal and Pathological Function.* Thorofare, NJ: Slack Incorporated.

Prince F, Winter DA, Stergiou P *et al.* (1994) Anticipatory control of upper body balance during human locomotion. *Gait and Posture* **2**: 19–25.

Prince F, Corriveau H, Hébert R *et al.* (1997) Gait in the elderly. *Gait and Posture* **5**: 128–135.

Radin EL. (1987) Osteoarthrosis: what is known about its prevention. *Clinical Orthopaedics and Related Research* **222**: 60–65.

Rose J, Gamble JG. (1994) *Human Walking,* 2nd edn. Baltimore, Maryland: Williams & Wilkins.

Sadeghi H. (2003) Local or global asymmetry in gait of people without impairments. *Gait and Posture* **17**: 197–204.

Saunders JBDM, Inman VT, Eberhart HS. (1953) The major determinants in normal and pathological gait. *Journal of Bone and Joint Surgery* **35A**: 543–558.

Sawatzky BJ, Sanderson DJ, Beauchamp RD *et al.* (1994) Ground reaction forces in gait in children with clubfeet – a preliminary study. *Gait and Posture* **2**: 123–127.

Sekiya N, Nagasaki H. (1998) Reproducibility of the walking patterns of normal young adults: test-retest reliability of the walk ratio (step-length/step-rate). *Gait and Posture* **7**: 225–227.

Shiavi R. (1985) Electromyographic patterns in adult locomotion: a comprehensive review. *Journal of Rehabilitation Research and Development* **22**: 85–98.

Siegel KL, Kepple TM, Stanhope SJ. (2004) Joint moment control of mechanical energy flow during normal gait. *Gait and Posture* **19**: 69–75.

Steindler A. (1953) A historical review of the studies and investigations made in relation to human gait. *Journal of Bone and Joint Surgery* **35A**: 540–542.

Sutherland DH. (1984) *Gait Disorders in Childhood and Adolescence*. Baltimore, MD: Williams & Wilkins.

Sutherland DH. (1997) The development of mature gait. *Gait and Posture* **6**: 163–170.

Sutherland DH. (2001) The evolution of clinical gait analysis. Part I: Kinesiological EMG. *Gait and Posture* **14**: 61–70.

Sutherland DH. (2002) The evolution of clinical gait analysis. Part II: Kinematics. *Gait and Posture* **16**: 159–1179.

Sutherland DH. (2005) The evolution of clinical gait analysis. Part III: Kinetics and energy assessment. *Gait and Posture* **21**: 447–461.

Sutherland DH, Olshen RA, Biden EN et al. (1988) *The Development of Mature Walking*. London: MacKeith Press.

Todd FN, Lamoreux LW, Skinner SR *et al.* (1989) Variations in the gait of normal children. *Journal of Bone and Joint Surgery* **71A**: 196–204.

Wall JC, Charteris J, Turnbull GI. (1987) Two steps equals one stride equals what?: the applicability of normal gait nomenclature to abnormal walking patterns. *Clinical Biomechanics* **2**: 119–125.

Waters RL, Mulroy S. (1999) The energy expenditure of normal and pathological gait. *Gait and Posture* **9**: 207–231.

Waters RL, Lunsford BR, Perry J *et al.* (1988) Energy–speed relationship of walking: standard tables. *Journal of Orthopaedic Research* **6**: 215–222.

Wells RP. (1981) The projection of the ground reaction force as a predictor of internal joint moments. *Bulletin of Prosthetic Research* **10–35**: 15–19.

Whittle MW. (1999) Generation and attenuation of transient impulsive forces beneath the foot: a review. *Gait and Posture* **10**: 264–275.

Winter DA. (1980) Overall principle of lower limb support during stance phase of gait. *Journal of Biomechanics* **13**: 923–927.

Winter DA. (1983) Energy generation and absorption at the ankle and knee during fast, natural and slow cadences. *Clinical Orthopaedics and Related Research* **175**: 147–154.

Winter DA. (1991) *The Biomechanics and Motor Control of Human Gait*, 2nd edn. Waterloo, Ontario: University of Waterloo Press.

Winter DA. (1995) Human balance and posture control during standing and walking. *Gait and Posture* **3**: 193–214.

Winter DA, Quanbury AO, Reimer GD. (1976) Analysis of instantaneous energy of normal gait. *Journal of Biomechanics* **9**: 253–257.

Pathological and other abnormal gaits

3

Although some variability is present in normal gait, particularly in the use of the muscles, there is an identifiable 'normal pattern' of walking and a 'normal range' can be defined for all of the variables which can be measured. Pathology of the locomotor system frequently produces gait patterns which are clearly 'abnormal'. Some of these abnormalities can be identified by eye, but others can only be identified by the use of appropriate measurement systems.

In order for a person to walk, the locomotor system must be able to accomplish four things:

1. Each leg in turn must be able to support the body weight without collapsing
2. Balance must be maintained, either statically or dynamically, during single leg stance
3. The swinging leg must be able to advance to a position where it can take over the supporting role
4. Sufficient power must be provided to make the necessary limb movements and to advance the trunk.

In normal walking, all of these are achieved without any apparent difficulty and with a modest energy consumption. However, in many forms of pathological gait they can be accomplished only by means of abnormal movements, which usually increase the energy consumption, or by the use of walking aids such as canes, crutches or orthoses (calipers and braces). If even one of these four requirements cannot be met, the subject is unable to walk.

The pattern of gait is the outcome of a complex interaction between the many neuromuscular and structural elements of the locomotor system. Abnormal gait may result from a disorder in any part of this system, including the brain, spinal cord, nerves, muscles, joints and skeleton. Abnormal gait may also result from the presence of pain, so that although a person is physically capable of walking normally, they find it more comfortable to walk in some other way.

The term *limp* is commonly used to describe a wide variety of abnormal gait patterns. However, dictionary definitions are unhelpful, a typical one being 'to walk lamely'. Since the word has no clearly defined scientific meaning, it should only be used with caution in the context of gait analysis. The most appropriate use of the word is probably for a gait abnormality involving some degree of asymmetry, which is readily apparent to an untrained observer.

Since gait is the end result of a complicated process, a number of different original problems may manifest themselves in the same abnormality of gait. For this reason, the abnormal gait patterns will be described separately from the pathological conditions which cause them. The first part of the chapter describes, in some detail, the most common abnormal gait patterns. This is followed by a description of the use of walking aids and the gait of amputees. The chapter ends with a description of the way in which gait abnormalities may result from a number of common but serious neurological conditions.

SPECIFIC GAIT ABNORMALITIES

The following section is based on a manual of lecture notes for student orthotists, published by New York University (1986). It includes a very useful list of common gait abnormalities, all of which can be identified by eye. The manual criticizes the common practice of identifying gait abnormalities by their pathological cause, for example 'hemiplegic gait', which immediately suggests that all hemiplegics walk in the same way, which is far from true, and also neglects the changes in gait which may occur with the passage of time, or result from treatment. The manual suggests that it is preferable to use purely descriptive terms, such as 'excessive medial foot contact'. This practice will be adopted in the following section. Some of the gait abnormalities described in the New York University publication applied only to the gait of subjects wearing orthoses; these descriptions have been omitted from the present text.

The pathological gait patterns to be described may occur either alone or in combination. If in combination, they may interact, so that the individual gait modifications do not exactly fit the description. The list that follows is not exhaustive; a subject may use a variation of one of the general patterns or may use another gait pattern which is not listed here.

When studying a pathological gait, particularly one which does not appear to fit into one of the standard patterns, it is helpful to remember that an abnormal movement may be performed for one of two reasons:

1. The subject has no choice, the movement being 'forced' on them by weakness, spasticity or deformity

2. The movement is a compensation, which the subject is using to correct for some other problem, which therefore needs to be identified.

Lateral trunk bending

Bending the trunk towards the side of the supporting limb during the stance phase is known as lateral trunk bending, ipsilateral lean or, more commonly, a *Trendelenburg gait*. The purpose of the maneuver is generally to reduce the forces in the abductor muscles and hip joint during single leg stance.

Lateral trunk bending is best observed from the front or the back. During the double support phase, the trunk is generally upright but as soon as the swing leg leaves the ground, the trunk leans over towards the side of the stance phase leg, returning to the upright attitude again at the beginning of the next double support phase. The trunk bending may unilateral, being restricted to the stance phase of one leg, or it may be bilateral, the trunk swaying from one side to the other, to produce a gait pattern known as *waddling*.

In the examples which follow, the weight of the trunk is 452 N, corresponding to a mass of 46 kg, and the weight of the right leg is 147 N, corresponding to a mass of 15 kg. As explained in Chapter 1 (p. 32), weight is a force, calculated by multiplying an object's mass by the acceleration due to gravity, 9.81 m/s².

Figure 3.1 shows a schematic of the trunk, pelvis and hip joints when standing on both legs. The abductor muscles are inactive and the weight of the trunk is divided equally between the two hip joints. Figure 3.2 shows what happens in a normal individual when the right foot is lifted off the ground: the force through the left hip joint increases by a factor of six, from 226 N (23 kgf or 51 lbf) to 1510 N (154 kgf or 339 lbf). This increase in force is made up of three components:

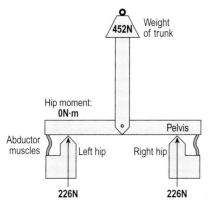

Fig. 3.1 Schematic of double legged stance: the force in each hip joint (226 N) is half the weight of the trunk (452 N). The abductors are not contracting.

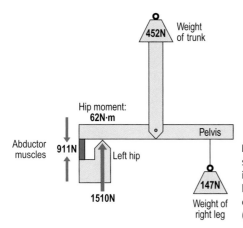

Fig. 3.2 Schematic of single legged stance. The force in the left hip (1510 N) is the sum of: a) weight of trunk (452 N), b) weight of right leg (147 N), and c) contraction force of abductor muscles (911 N).

1. The whole of the weight of the trunk is now supported by the left hip joint, instead of being shared between the two hips
2. The weight of the right leg is now taken by the left hip, instead of by the ground
3. The left hip abductors (primarily gluteus medius) contract, producing an anticlockwise moment to keep the pelvis from dropping on the unsupported side. The reaction force to this contraction passes through the left hip.

These three components contribute to the increased force in the left hip as follows:

1. Trunk weight not shared: 226 N (23 kgf or 51 lbf)
2. Weight of right leg: 147 N (15 kgf or 33 lbf)
3. Contraction of abductors: 911 N (93 kgf or 204 lbf)
Total: 1284 N (131 kgf or 288 lbf).

It should be noted that this example was invented for the purposes of illustration – the actual numbers should not be taken too seriously!

The four conditions which must be met if this mechanism is to operate satisfactorily are:

1. The absence of significant pain on loading
2. Adequate power in the hip abductors
3. A sufficiently long lever arm for the hip abductors
4. A solid and stable fulcrum in or around the hip joint.

Should one or more of these conditions not be met, the subject may adopt lateral trunk bending in an attempt to compensate.

The effect of lateral trunk bending on the joint force is shown in Fig. 3.3. There is no effect on components (1) and (2) of the increased force, but

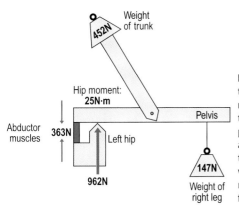

Fig. 3.3 Lateral trunk bending: bringing the trunk across the supporting hip reduces the clockwise moments about the left hip from 62 N·m to 25 N·m, permitting the pelvis to be stabilized by a smaller abductor force. The force in the left hip (962 N) is the sum of: a) weight of trunk (452 N), b) weight of right leg (147 N), and c) contraction force of abductor muscles (363 N).

if the center of gravity of the trunk is moved directly above the left hip, this eliminates the clockwise moment produced by the mass of the trunk. The abductors are now only required to contract with a force of 363 N (37 kgf or 81 lbf) to balance the clockwise moment provided by the weight of the right leg. There is thus a reduction of 548 N (56 kgf or 123 lbf) in the abductor contraction force and a corresponding reduction in the total joint force, from 1501 N down to 962 N. The numbers in the illustrations refer to standing; during the stance phase of walking, higher forces are to be expected due to the vertical accelerations of the center of gravity, which cause the force transmitted through the leg to fluctuate above and below body weight (see Fig. 2.19). However, these fluctuations tend to be less in pathological than in normal gait, since the vertical accelerations are less in someone walking with a shorter stride length. The numbers also suppose that the bending of the trunk brings its center of gravity exactly above the hip joint. This is unlikely to happen in practice, of course, but the principles remain the same, whether the center of gravity is not deviated as far as the hip joint or even if it passes lateral to it.

There are a number of conditions in which this gait abnormality is adopted.

1. Painful hip: If the hip joint is painful, as in osteoarthritis and rheumatoid arthritis, the amount of pain experienced usually depends to a very large extent on the force being transmitted through the joint. Since lateral trunk bending reduces the total joint force, 'Trendelenburg gait' is extremely common in people with arthritis of the hip. Although it produces a useful reduction in force and hence in pain, the forces still remain substantial (962 N in Fig. 3.3) and some form of definitive treatment is usually required.

2. Hip abductor weakness: If the hip abductors are weak, they may be unable to contract with sufficient force to stabilize the pelvis during single leg stance. In this case, the pelvis will dip on the side of the foot which is off the ground (Trendelenburg's sign, as opposed to 'Trendelenburg gait'). In order to reduce the demands on the weakened muscles, the subject will usually employ lateral trunk bending, in both standing and walking, to reduce joint moment as far as possible (Fig. 3.4). Hip abductor weakness may be caused by disease or injury affecting either the muscles themselves or the nervous system which controls them.

3. Abnormal hip joint: Three conditions around the hip joint will lead to difficulties in stabilizing the pelvis using the abductors: congenital dislocation of the hip (CDH, also known as developmental dysplasia of the hip), coxa vara and slipped femoral epiphysis. In all three, the effective length of the gluteus medius is reduced because the greater trochanter of the femur moves proximally, towards the pelvic brim. Since the muscle is shortened, it is unable to function efficiently and thus contracts with a reduced tension. In CDH and severe cases of slipped femoral epiphysis, a further problem exists in that the normal hip joint is effectively lost, to be replaced by a false hip joint, or pseudarthrosis. This abnormal joint is more laterally placed, giving a reduced lever arm for the abductor muscles, and it may fail to provide the 'solid and stable fulcrum' mentioned above (p. 104). The combination of reduced lever arm and reduced muscle force gives these subjects a powerful incentive to walk with lateral trunk bending (Fig. 3.5). In many cases, particularly in older people with CDH, the false hip joint becomes arthritic and they add a painful hip to their other problems. Pain is frequently also a factor in slipped femoral epiphysis.

4. Wide walking base: If the walking base is abnormally wide, there is a problem with balance during single leg stance. Rather than tip the whole body to maintain balance, as in Fig. 2.27a, lateral bending of the trunk may be used to keep the center of gravity of the body roughly over the supporting leg. In most cases, this will need to be done during the stance phase on both sides, leading to bilateral trunk bending and a waddling gait. A number of conditions, which will be described later, may cause a wide walking base.

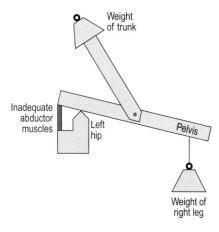

Weight of trunk

Inadequate abductor muscles

Left hip

Pelvis

Weight of right leg

Fig. 3.4 Trendelenburg's sign: due to inadequate hip abductors, the pelvis drops on the unsupported side when one foot is lifted off the ground. To compensate, the subject bends the trunk over the supporting hip.

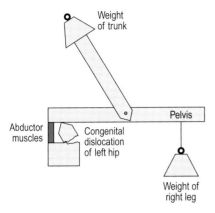

Fig. 3.5 Congenital dislocation of the hip (CDH): both the working length and the lever arm of the hip abductors are reduced. To compensate, the subject bends the trunk over the supporting hip.

5. Unequal leg length: When walking with an unequal leg length, the pelvis tips downwards on the side of the shortened limb, as the body weight is transferred to it. This is sometimes described as 'stepping into a hole'. The pelvic tilt is accompanied by a compensatory lateral bend of the trunk.

6. Other causes: Perry (1992) gives a number of other causes for lateral bending of the trunk, including adductor contracture, scoliosis and an impaired body image, typically following a stroke.

Anterior trunk bending

In anterior trunk bending, the subject flexes his or her trunk forwards early in the stance phase. If only one leg is affected, the trunk is straightened again around the time of opposite initial contact, but if both sides are affected, the trunk may be kept flexed throughout the gait cycle. This gait abnormality is best seen from the side.

One important purpose of this gait pattern is to compensate for an inadequacy of the knee extensors. The left diagram of Fig. 3.6 shows that early in the stance phase, the line of action of the ground reaction force vector normally passes behind the axis of the knee joint and generates an external moment which attempts to flex it. This is opposed by contraction of the quadriceps, to generate an internal extension moment. If the quadriceps is weak or paralyzed, it cannot generate this internal moment and the knee will tend to collapse. As shown in the right-hand diagram of Fig. 3.6, anterior trunk bending is used to move the center of gravity of the body forwards, which results in the line of force passing in front of the axis of the knee, producing an external extension (or hyperextension) moment. In addition to anterior trunk bending, subjects will sometimes keep one hand on the affected thigh while walking, to provide further stabilization for the knee.

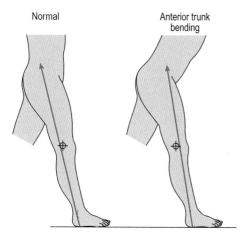

Normal

Anterior trunk
bending

Fig. 3.6 Anterior trunk bending: in normal walking, the line of force early in the stance phase passes behind the knee; anterior trunk bending brings the line of force in front of the knee, to compensate for weak knee extensors.

Other causes for anterior trunk bending are equinus deformity of the foot, hip extensor weakness and hip flexion contracture (Perry, 1992).

Posterior trunk bending

One form of posterior trunk bending is essentially a reversed version of anterior trunk bending, in that early in the stance phase, the whole trunk moves in the sagittal plane, but this time backwards instead of forwards. Again, it is most easily observed from the side. The purpose of this is to compensate for ineffective hip extensors. The line of the ground reaction force early in the stance phase normally passes in front of the hip joint (Fig. 3.7, left). This produces an external moment which attempts to flex the trunk forward on the thigh, opposed by contraction of the hip extensors, particularly gluteus maximus. Should these muscles be weak or paralyzed, the subject may compensate by moving the trunk backwards at this time, bringing the line of action of the external force behind the axis of the hip joint, as shown in the right-hand diagram of Fig. 3.7.

A different type of posterior trunk bending may occur early in the swing phase, where the subject may throw the trunk backwards in order to propel the swinging leg forwards. This is most often used to compensate for weakness of the hip flexors or spasticity of the hip extensors, either of which makes it difficult to accelerate the femur forwards at the beginning of swing. This maneuver may also be used if the knee is unable to flex, since the whole leg must be accelerated forwards as one unit, which greatly increases the demands on the hip flexors. Posterior trunk bending may also occur when the hip is ankylosed (fused), the trunk moving backwards as the thigh moves forwards.

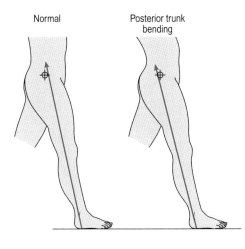

Normal

Posterior trunk
bending

Fig. 3.7 Posterior trunk bending: in normal walking, the line of force early in the stance phase passes in front of the hip; posterior trunk bending brings the line of force behind the hip, to compensate for weak hip extensors.

Increased lumbar lordosis

Many people have an exaggerated lumbar lordosis, but it is only regarded as a gait abnormality if the lordosis is used to aid walking in some way, which generally means that the degree of lordosis varies during the course of the gait cycle. Increased lumbar lordosis is observed from the side of the subject and generally reaches a peak at the end of the stance phase on the affected side.

The most common cause of increased lumbar lordosis is a flexion contracture of the hip. It is also seen if the hip joint is immobile due to ankylosis. Both of these deformities cause the stride length to be very short, by preventing the femur from moving backwards from its flexed position. This difficulty can be overcome if the femur can be brought into the vertical (or even extended) position, not through movement at the hip joint but by extension of the lumbar spine, with a consequent increase in the lumbar lordosis (Fig. 3.8).

The orientation of the pelvis in the sagittal plane is maintained by the opposing pulls of the trunk muscles above and the limb muscles below. If there is muscle imbalance, for example a weakness of the muscles of the anterior abdominal wall, weakness of the hip extensors or spasticity of the hip flexors, the subject may develop an excessive *anterior pelvic tilt*, again with an increase in the lumbar lordosis.

Functional leg length discrepancy

Four gait abnormalities (circumduction, hip hiking, steppage and vaulting) are closely related, in that they are designed to overcome the same problem – a functional discrepancy in leg length. A review on the topic of leg length discrepancy was published by Gurney (2002).

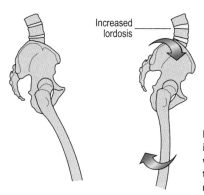

Increased
lordosis

Fig. 3.8 Increased lumbar lordosis: when there is a fixed flexion deformity of the hip (left), the whole pelvis must rotate forwards for the femur to move into a vertical position (right), with a resulting increase in lumbar lordosis.

An 'anatomical' leg length discrepancy occurs when the legs are actually different lengths, as measured with a tape measure or, more accurately, by long-leg x-rays. A 'functional' leg length discrepancy means that the legs are not necessarily different lengths (although they may be) but that one or both are unable to adjust to the appropriate length for a particular phase of the gait cycle. In order for natural walking to occur, the stance phase leg needs to be longer than the swing phase leg. If it is not, the swinging leg collides with the ground and is unable to pass the stance leg. The way that a leg is functionally lengthened (for the stance phase) is to extend at the hip and knee and to plantarflex at the ankle. Conversely, the way in which a leg is functionally shortened (for the swing phase) is to flex at the hip and knee and to dorsiflex at the ankle. Failure to achieve all the necessary flexions and extensions is likely to lead to a functional leg discrepancy and hence to one of these gait abnormalities. This usually occurs as the result of a neurological problem. Spasticity of any of the extensors or weakness of any of the flexors tends to make a leg too long in the swing phase, as does the mechanical locking of a joint in extension. Conversely, spasticity of the flexors, weakness of the extensors or a flexion contracture in a joint makes the limb too short for the stance phase. Other causes of functional leg length discrepancy include musculoskeletal problems such as sacroiliac joint dysfunction.

An increase in functional leg length is particularly common following a 'stroke', where a foot drop (due to anterior tibial weakness or paralysis) may be accompanied by an increase in tone in the hip and knee extensor muscles.

The gait modifications designed to overcome the problem may either lengthen the stance phase leg or shorten the swing phase leg, thus allowing a normal swing to occur. They are not mutually exclusive and a subject may use them in combination. The gait modification employed by a particular person may have been forced on them by the underlying pathology or it may have been a matter of chance, two people with apparently identical clinical conditions having found different solutions to the problem.

Circumduction

Ground contact by the swinging leg can be avoided if it is swung outward, in a movement known as circumduction (Fig. 3.9). The swing phase of the other leg will usually be normal. The movement of circumduction is best seen from in front or behind.

Circumduction may also be used to advance the swinging leg in the presence of weak hip flexors, by improving the ability of the adductor muscles to act as hip flexors while the hip joint is extended.

Hip hiking

Hip hiking is a gait modification in which the pelvis is lifted on the side of the swinging leg (Fig. 3.10), by contraction of the spinal muscles and the lateral abdominal wall. The movement is best seen from behind or in front.

By tipping the pelvis up on the side of the swinging leg, hip hiking involves a reversal of the second determinant of gait (pelvic obliquity about an anteroposterior axis). It may also involve an exaggeration of the first determinant (pelvic rotation about a vertical axis), to assist with leg advancement. Leg advancement may also be helped by posterior trunk bending at the beginning of the swing phase.

According to the manual by New York University (1986), hip hiking is commonly used in slow walking with weak hamstrings, since the knee tends to extend prematurely and thus to make the leg too long towards the end of the swing phase. It is seldom employed for limb lengthening due to plantarflexion of the ankle.

Steppage

Steppage is a very simple swing phase modification, consisting of exaggerated knee and hip flexion, to lift the foot higher than usual for increased ground

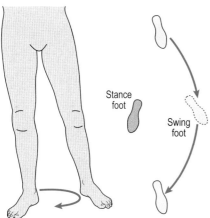

Fig. 3.9 Circumduction: the swinging leg moves in an arc, rather than straight forwards, to increase the ground clearance for the swing foot.

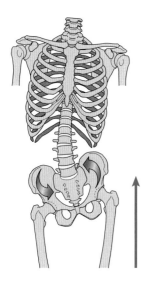

Fig. 3.10 Hip hiking: the swing phase leg is lifted by raising the pelvis on that side.

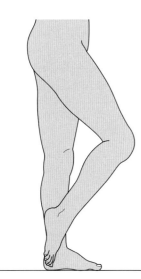

Fig. 3.11 Steppage: increased hip and knee flexion improve ground clearance for the swing phase leg, in this case necessitated by a foot drop.

clearance (Fig. 3.11). It is best observed from the side.

It is particularly used to compensate for a plantarflexed ankle, commonly known as *foot drop*, due to inadequate dorsiflexion control, which will be described later.

Vaulting

The ground clearance for the swinging leg will be increased if the subject goes up on the toes of the stance phase leg, a movement known as vaulting (Fig. 3.12). This causes an exaggerated vertical movement of the trunk, which is both ungainly in appearance and wasteful of energy. It may be observed from either the side or the front.

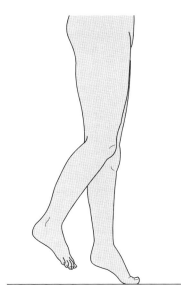

Fig. 3.12 Vaulting: the subject goes up on the toes of the stance phase leg to increase ground clearance for the swing phase leg.

Vaulting is a stance phase modification, whereas the related gait abnormalities (circumduction, hip hiking and steppage) are swing phase modifications. For this reason, vaulting may be a more appropriate solution for problems involving the swing phase leg. Like hip hiking, it is commonly used in slow walking with hamstring weakness, when the knee tends to extend too early in the swing phase. It may also be used on the 'normal' side of an above-knee amputee whose prosthetic knee fails to flex adequately in the swing phase.

Abnormal hip rotation

Because the hip is able to make large rotations in the transverse plane, for which the knee and ankle cannot compensate, an abnormal rotation at the hip involves the whole leg, with the foot showing an abnormal 'toe in' or 'toe out' alignment. The gait pattern may involve both stance and swing phases and is best observed from behind or in front.

Abnormal hip rotation may result from one of three causes:

1. A problem with the muscles producing hip rotation
2. A fault in the way the foot makes contact with the ground
3. As a compensatory movement to overcome some other problem.

Problems with the muscles producing hip rotation usually involve spasticity or weakness of the muscles which rotate the femur about the hip joint. For example, overactivity of the hip extensors in cerebral palsy may include an element of internal rotation. Imbalance between the medial and lateral hamstrings is a common cause of rotation; weakness of biceps femoris or spasticity of the medial hamstrings will cause internal rotation of the leg. Conversely, spasticity of biceps femoris or weakness of the medial hamstrings will result in an external rotation.

A number of foot disorders will produce an abnormal rotation at the hip. Inversion of the foot, whether due to a fixed inversion (pes varus) or to weakness of the peroneal muscles, will internally rotate the whole limb when weight is taken on it. A corresponding eversion of the foot, whether fixed (pes valgus) or due to weakness of the anterior and posterior tibial muscles, will result in an external rotation of the leg.

External rotation may be used as a compensation for quadriceps weakness, to alter the direction of the line of force through the knee. This could be used as an alternative to, or in addition to, anterior trunk bending. External rotation may also be used to facilitate hip flexion, using the adductors as flexors, if the true hip flexors are weak. Subjects with weakness of the triceps surae may also externally rotate the leg, to permit the use of the peroneal muscles as plantar flexors.

Excessive knee extension

In the gait abnormality of excessive knee extension, the normal stance phase flexion of the knee is lost, to be replaced by full extension or even hyperextension, in which the knee is angulated backwards. This is best seen from the side.

One cause of knee hyperextension has already been described: quadriceps weakness can be compensated for by keeping the leg fully extended, using anterior trunk bending (Fig. 3.6), external rotation of the leg, or both, to keep the line of the ground reaction force from passing behind the axis of the knee joint. Other means of keeping the knee fully extended are pushing the thigh back by keeping one hand on it while walking and using the hip extensors to snap the thigh sharply back at the time of initial contact.

Hyperextension of the knee, accompanied by anterior trunk bending, is seen quite frequently in people with paralysis of the quadriceps following poliomyelitis. The gait abnormality is clearly of great value to the subject, since without it he or she would be unable to walk. However, the external hyperextension moment is resisted by tension in the posterior joint capsule, which gradually stretches, allowing the knee to develop a hyperextension deformity ('genu recurvatum'). As a result of this deformity, the joint frequently develops osteoarthritis in later life.

This is illustrated in Fig. 3.13, which shows the left sagittal plane hip, knee and ankle angles during walking in a 41-year-old woman, whose quadriceps were paralyzed on both sides by poliomyelitis at the age of 12. She walked very

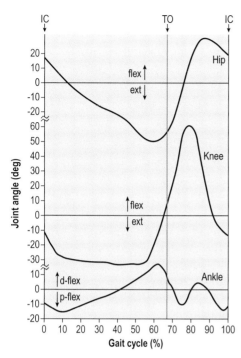

Fig. 3.13 Excessive knee extension: sagittal plane hip, knee and ankle angles in a subject with paralyzed quadriceps, showing gross hyperextension of the knee and increased extension of the hip. Abbreviations as in Fig. 2.5.

slowly, using two forearm crutches (cycle time 1.9 s; cadence 63 steps/min; stride length 1.00 m; speed 0.52 m/s). The knee hyperextended to 32° during weightbearing, but flexed normally to 63° during the swing phase. The hip extended more than in normal individuals, since hyperextension of the knee places the knee joint more posteriorly than usual, thus altering the angle of the femur.

In normal walking, an external moment attempts to hyperextend the knee during terminal stance. This is resisted by an internal flexor moment (see Fig. 2.6), generated primarily by gastrocnemius. Should gastrocnemius be weak, the knee may be pushed backwards into hyperextension. This may help with walking, since the leg lengthening required during pre-swing can be provided by extending the knee, rather than by plantarflexing the ankle. However, there is a risk that the knee will go beyond full extension into hyperextension, with consequent damage to the posterior capsule.

Hyperextension of the knee is common in spasticity. One common cause is overactivity of the quadriceps, which extends the knee directly. Another is spasticity of the triceps surae, which plantarflexes the ankle and causes the body weight to be taken through the forefoot. The resulting forward displacement of the ground reaction force vector generates an external moment which is an exaggeration of the normal 'plantarflexion/knee extension couple' and results in hyperextension of the knee.

Shortness of one leg may cause a person, when standing, to take all their weight on the other (longer) leg, with the knee hyperextended. This is because it is uncomfortable to stand on both legs, since the knee on the longer side would have to be kept flexed.

Excessive knee flexion

The knee is normally fully extended (or nearly so) twice during the gait cycle: around initial contact and around heel rise. In the gait abnormality known as excessive knee flexion, one or both of these movements into extension fails to occur. The flexion and extension of the knee are best seen from the side of the subject.

A flexion contracture of the knee will obviously prevent it from extending normally. A flexion contracture of the hip may also prevent the knee from extending, if hip flexion prevents the femur from becoming vertical or extended during the latter part of the stance phase (Fig. 3.14). By reducing the effective length of the leg during the stance phase, one of the compensations for a functional discrepancy in leg length will probably also be required.

Spasticity of the knee flexors may also cause the gait pattern of excessive knee flexion. Since the knee flexors are able to overpower the quadriceps, this may lead to other gait modifications, such as anterior trunk bending, to compensate for a relative weakness of the quadriceps.

The knee may flex excessively following initial contact if the normal plantarflexion of the foot during loading response is prevented, through immobility of the ankle joint or a calcaneus deformity of the foot, preventing the force vector from migrating forwards along the foot.

Increased flexion of the knee may also be part of a compensatory movement, either to reduce the effective limb length in functional leg length

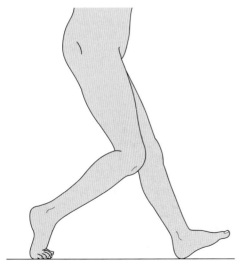

Fig. 3.14 Excessive knee flexion: in late stance phase there is increased knee flexion, caused by a flexion contracture of the hip.

discrepancy or as part of a pattern of exaggerated hip, knee and arm movements, to make up for a lack of plantarflexor power in push off.

Inadequate dorsiflexion control

The dorsiflexors are active at two different times during the gait cycle, so inadequate dorsiflexion control may give rise to two different gait abnormalities. During loading response, the dorsiflexors resist the external plantarflexion moment, thus permitting the foot to be lowered to the ground gently. If they are weak, the foot is lowered abruptly in a *foot slap*. The dorsiflexors are also active during the swing phase, when they are used to raise the foot and achieve ground clearance. Failure to raise the foot sufficiently during initial swing may cause *toe drag*. Both problems are best observed from the side of the subject and both make a distinctive noise. A subject with inadequate dorsiflexion control can often be diagnosed by ear, before they have come into view!

Inadequate dorsiflexion control may result from weakness or paralysis of the anterior tibial muscles or from these muscles being overpowered by spasticity of the triceps surae. An inability to dorsiflex the foot during the swing phase causes a functional leg length discrepancy, for which a number of compensations were described previously. Toe drag will only be observed if the subject fails to compensate. Toe drag may also occur if there is delayed flexion of the hip or knee in initial swing, causing the foot to catch on the ground, despite adequate dorsiflexion at the ankle.

Even if they suffer from inadequate dorsiflexion control, subjects with spasticity are frequently able to achieve dorsiflexion in the swing phase, because flexion of the hip and knee are often accompanied by reflex dorsiflexion of the ankle, in a primitive movement pattern related to the flexor withdrawal reflex, mentioned in Chapter 1 (p. 30).

Abnormal foot contact

The foot may be abnormally loaded so that the weight is primarily borne on only one of its four quadrants. Loading on the heel or forefoot is best observed from the side and loading on the medial or lateral side is best observed from the front, although some authorities state that the foot should always be observed from behind. Where a glass walkway is available, viewing the foot from below gives an excellent idea of the pattern of foot loading.

Loading of the heel occurs in the deformity known as *talipes calcaneus* (also known as pes calcaneus), where the forefoot is pulled up into extreme dorsiflexion (Fig. 3.15), usually as a result of muscle imbalance, such as

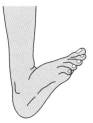

Fig. 3.15 Talipes calcaneus.

results from spasticity of the anterior tibial muscles or weakness of the triceps surae. Except in mild cases, weight is never taken by the forefoot and the stance phase duration is reduced by the loss of the 'terminal rocker' (p. 91). The reduced stance phase duration on the affected side reduces the swing phase duration on the opposite side, which in turn reduces the opposite step length and the overall stride length. The ground reaction force vector remains posterior, producing an increased external flexion moment at the knee.

In the deformity known as *talipes equinus* (or pes equinus) (Fig. 3.16), the forefoot is fixed in plantarflexion, usually through spasticity of the plantarflexors. In a mild equinus deformity, the foot may be placed onto the ground flat; in more severe cases the heel never contacts the ground at all and initial contact is made by the metatarsal heads, in a gait pattern known as *primary toestrike*. Because the line of force from the ground reaction is displaced anteriorly, an increased external moment tending to extend the knee is present (plantarflexion/knee extension couple). The loss of the initial rocker (p. 91) shortens the stride length.

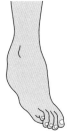

Fig. 3.16 Talipes equinus.

Excessive medial contact occurs in a number of foot deformities. Weakness of the inverters or spasticity of the everters will cause the medial side of the foot to drop and to take most of the weight. In *pes valgus*, the medial arch is lowered, permitting weight bearing on the medial border of the foot. Increased medial foot contact may also be due to a valgus deformity of the knee, accompanied by an increased walking base.

Excessive lateral foot contact may also result from foot deformity, when the medial border of the foot is elevated or the lateral border depressed, by

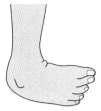

Fig. 3.17 Talipes equinovarus.

spasticity or weakness. The foot deformity known as *talipes equinovarus* (Fig. 3.17) combines equinus with varus, producing a curved foot where all the load is borne by the outer border of the forefoot. Although the term *club foot* may be applied to any foot deformity, it is most commonly applied to talipes equinovarus.

Another form of abnormal foot contact is the *stamping* that commonly accompanies a loss of sensation in the foot, such as occurs in tabes dorsalis, the final stage of syphilis. The subject receives feedback on ground contact from the vibration caused by the impact of the foot on the ground.

Abnormal foot rotation

Normal individuals place the foot on the ground approximately in line with the direction of walk, typically with a few degrees of toe out. Pathological toe in or toe out angles may be produced by internal or external hip rotation, torsion (twisting) of the femur or tibia, or deformity of the foot itself. An important consequence of an abnormal foot rotation is that it causes the ground reaction force to be in an abnormal position relative to the rest of the leg. For example, if the foot is internally rotated, the ground reaction force is more medial than normal, which will generate external adductor moments at the ankle and knee. In either internal or external foot rotation, the effective length of the foot is reduced in the direction of progression, so that the ground reaction force during terminal stance and pre-swing is likely to be more posterior than normal. This reduces the lever arm for the triceps surae to generate an internal plantarflexion moment.

This is one example of a problem known as *lever arm disease* or *lever arm deficiency*, in which individuals with normal muscle strength are unable to generate sufficient internal joint moments, due to a reduction in the length of a muscle's lever arm. This is particularly seen in individuals with cerebral palsy who have a severe degree of internal or external foot rotation; the resulting posterior placement of the ground reaction force increases the external moment flexing the knee.

Insufficient push off

In normal walking, weight is borne on the forefoot during the 'push off' in pre-swing. In the gait pattern known as insufficient push off, the weight is taken primarily on the heel and there is no push off phase, the whole foot being lifted off the ground at once. It is best observed from the side.

The main cause of insufficient push off is a problem with the triceps surae or Achilles tendon, which prevents adequate weight bearing on the forefoot. Rupture of the Achilles tendon and weakness of the soleus and gastrocnemius are typical causes. Weakness or paralysis of the intrinsic muscles of the foot may also prevent the foot from taking load through the forefoot.

Insufficient push off may also result from any foot deformity, if the anatomy is so distorted that it prevents normal forefoot loading. A calcaneus deformity (Fig. 3.15) obviously makes it impossible to put any significant load on the forefoot.

Another important cause of insufficient push off is pain under the forefoot, if the amount of pain is affected by the degree of loading (as it usually is). This may occur in metatarsalgia and also when arthritis affects the metatarsophalangeal joints. The loss of the terminal rocker causes the foot to leave the ground prematurely, before the hip has fully extended. This reduces the stance phase duration on the affected side and hence the swing phase duration and step length on the opposite side, and produces an asymmetry in gait timing.

Abnormal walking base

The walking base is usually in the range 50–130mm. In pathological gait it may be either increased or decreased beyond this range. While ideally determined by actual measurement, changes in the walking base may be estimated by eye, preferably from behind the subject.

An increased walking base may be caused by any deformity, such as an abducted hip or valgus knee, which causes the feet to be placed on the ground wider apart than usual. A consequence of an increased walking base is that increased lateral movement of the trunk is required to maintain balance, as shown in Fig. 2.27.

The other important cause of an increased walking base is instability and a fear of falling, the feet being placed wide apart to increase the area of support. This allows a margin of error in the positioning of the center of gravity over the feet. This gait abnormality is likely to be present when there is a deficiency in the sensation or proprioception of the legs, so that the subject is not quite sure where the feet are, relative to the trunk. It is also used in cerebellar ataxia, to increase the level of security in an uncoordinated gait pattern. Another effective way to improve stability is to walk with one or two canes.

A narrow walking base usually results from an adduction deformity at the hip or a varus deformity at the knee. Hip adduction may cause the swing phase leg to cross the midline, in a gait pattern known as *scissoring*, which is commonly seen in cerebral palsy. In milder cases, the swing phase leg is able to pass the stance phase leg, but then moves across in front of it. In more severe cases, the swinging leg is unable to pass the stance leg: it stops behind it, with the side-to-side positions of the two feet reversed. This is clearly a very disabling gait pattern, with a very short stride length and negative values for the walking base and for the step length on one side.

Rhythmic disturbances

Gait disorders may include abnormalities in the timing of the gait cycle. Two types of rhythmic disturbance can be identified: an *asymmetric* rhythmic disturbance shows a difference in the gait timing between the two legs; an *irregular* rhythmic disturbance shows differences between one stride and the next. Rhythmic disturbances are best observed from the side and may also be audible.

An *antalgic* gait pattern is specifically a gait modification which reduces the amount of pain a person is experiencing. The term is usually applied to a rhythmic disturbance, in which as short a time as possible is spent on the painful limb and a correspondingly longer time is spent on the pain-free side. The pattern is asymmetrical between the two legs but is generally regular from one cycle to the next. A marked difference in leg length between the two sides may also produce a regular gait asymmetry of this type, as may a number of other differences between the two sides, such as joint contractures or ankylosis.

Irregular gait rhythmic disturbances, where the timing alters from one step to the next, are seen in a number of neurological conditions. In particular, cerebellar ataxia leads to loss of the 'pattern generator', responsible for a regular, coordinated sequence of footsteps. Loss of sensation or proprioception may also cause an irregular arrhythmia, due to a general uncertainty about limb position and orientation.

Other gait abnormalities

A number of other gait abnormalities may be observed, either alone or in combination with some of the gait patterns described above. They include:

1. Abnormal movements, for example intention tremors and athetoid movements
2. Abnormal attitude or movements of the upper limb, including a failure to swing the arms
3. Abnormal attitude or movements of the head and neck
4. Sideways rotation of the foot following heelstrike
5. Excessive external rotation of the foot during swing, sometimes called a 'whip'
6. Rapid fatigue.

This account has concentrated on gait abnormalities which may be observed visually. However, a number of gait abnormalities can only be detected using kinetic/kinematic gait analysis systems. An example is the presence of an abnormal moment, such as the excessive internal varus moment which may be present in the knee of children with myelomeningocele and which may predispose them to the development of osteoarthritis (Lim *et al.*, 1998).

WALKING AIDS

The use of walking aids may modify the gait pattern considerably. While some people choose to use a walking aid to make it easier to walk, for example to reduce the pain in a painful joint, others are totally unable to walk without some form of aid. Although there are many detailed variations in design, walking aids, also called 'assistive devices', can be classified into three basic types – *canes*, *crutches* and *frames*. All three operate by supporting part of the body weight through the arm rather than the leg. While this is an effective way of coping with inadequacies of the legs, it frequently leads to problems with the wrist and shoulder joints, which are simply not designed for the transmission of large forces.

There is considerable variability in the way in which walking aids are used and people will often use them in ways which do not quite fit the typical patterns described in the following sections.

Canes

The simplest form of walking aid is the cane, also known as a walking stick, by means of which force can be transmitted to the ground through the wrist and hand. Since the forearm muscles are relatively weak and the joints of the wrist fairly small, it is impossible to transmit large forces through a cane for any length of time. The torque which can be applied to the upper end of the cane is limited by the grip strength and by the shape of the handle, since the hand tends to slip. For this reason the major direction of force transmission is along the axis of the cane. Canes may be used for three purposes, which are often combined:

1. To improve stability
2. To generate a moment
3. To take part of the load away from one of the legs.

1. Improve stability: Canes are frequently used by the elderly and infirm to improve their stability. This is achieved by increasing the size of the area of support, thus removing the need to position the center of gravity over the relatively small supporting area provided by the feet. In those with only minor stability problems, a single cane may be used. This will not provide a secure supporting area during single limb support, but does make it easier to correct for small imbalances. Since the cane is usually placed on the ground some distance away from the feet, giving a relatively long lever arm, a modest force through the cane will produce a substantial moment to correct for any positioning error. For maximum security, a person will need to use two canes, so that a triangular supporting area is always available. This is provided by two canes and one foot during single limb support and by one cane and two feet during double support. If only a single cane is used, it will normally be advanced during the stance phase of the more secure leg. If two canes are used, they are usually advanced separately, during double limb support, to provide the maximum stability at all times.

2. Generate a moment: The use of a cane to generate a moment is illustrated in Fig. 3.18. This should be compared with Fig. 3.2, which shows the mechanics of normal single legged stance. A vertical force of 100 N (10 kgf or 22 lbf) is applied through the cane, which generates a counterclockwise moment, applied to the shoulder girdle and hence to the pelvis. This reduces the size of the moment which the hip abductor muscles need to generate to keep the pelvis level. The contraction of these muscles is reduced from 911 N (93 kgf or 204 lbf) to 463 N (47 kgf or 104 lbf), a reduction of 448 N (56 kgf or 123 lbf). The total force in the hip joint is reduced by the sum of this amount and the force applied by the cane to the ground. For this mechanism to work, the cane must be held in the opposite hand to the painful hip. A cane may also be used to generate a lateral moment at the knee, to reduce the loading on one side of the joint. The cane is advanced during the swing phase of the leg it is protecting.

3. Reduce limb loading: When using a cane to remove some of the load from the leg, it is usually held in the same hand as the affected leg and placed on the ground close to the foot. In this way, load sharing can be achieved between the leg and the cane, even to the extent of removing the load entirely from the leg. The cane follows the movements of the affected leg, being advanced during

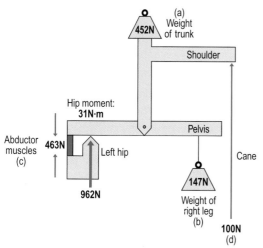

Fig. 3.18 The use of a cane to generate a counterclockwise moment reduces the contraction force of the hip abductors and hence the force in the hip joint. The force in the left hip (962 N) is the sum of: a) weight of trunk (452 N), b) weight of right leg (147 N), c) contraction force of abductor muscles (463 N), less: d) force through cane (100 N). (Compare with Fig. 3.2.)

the swing phase on that side. The person will normally lean sideways over the cane, in a lateral lurch, to increase the vertical loading on it and hence to reduce the load in the leg. A cane may be used in this way to relieve pain in the hip, knee, ankle or foot. If the cane is held in the opposite hand, as is often recommended, the lateral lurching can be avoided but the degree of off-loading is reduced.

Whichever of these three reasons a person has for using a cane, the degree of disability will determine whether one or two canes are used. It may be observed that a subject uses a cane in the opposite hand from what might have been expected. In some cases he or she has simply not discovered that they would benefit more from using the cane in the other hand but more often, the observer has failed to appreciate fully all the compensations which the subject has adopted.

There are a number of ways in which the simple cane can be modified, including many different types of handgrip. A particularly important variant on the simple cane is the *broad based cane*, also known as a *Hemi* or *crab cane*, which may have three feet (*tripod*) or four feet (*tetrapod* or *quad cane*). This differs from the simple cane in that it will stand up by itself and will tolerate small horizontal force components, so long as the overall force vector remains within the area of its base. It is particularly helpful when standing up from the sitting position. The increased stability is gained at the expense of an increase in weight and particularly bulk, which may cause difficulties when going through doorways.

Crutches

The main difference in function between a crutch and a cane is that a crutch is able to transmit significant forces in the horizontal plane. This is because, unlike the cane, which is effectively fixed to the body at only a single point, the crutch has two points of attachment, one at the hand and one higher up the arm, which provide a lever arm for the transmission of torque. Although there are many different designs of crutch, they fall into two categories: axillary crutches and forearm crutches. As with the cane, it is also possible to have a broad based crutch, ending in three or four feet.

Axillary crutches (Fig. 3.19 left), as their name suggests, fit under the axilla (armpit). They are usually of simple design, with a padded top surface and a hand-hold in the appropriate position. The lever arm between the axilla and the hand is fairly long and enough horizontal force can be generated to permit walking when both legs are straight and non-functional. A disadvantage of this type of crutch is that the axilla is not an ideal area for weight bearing and incorrect fitting or prolonged use may cause damage to the blood vessels or nerves. Although some people use axillary crutches for many years, they are more suitable for short-term use, for instance while a patient has a broken leg set in plaster.

There are many different types of *forearm crutches*, also called *elbow, Lofstrand* or *Canadian crutches* (Fig. 3.19 center). They differ from axillary

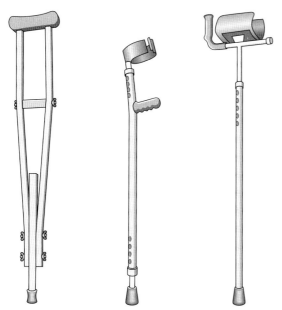

Fig. 3.19 Three types of crutch: axillary (left); forearm (center) and gutter (right).

crutches in that the upper point of contact between the body and the crutch is provided by either the forearm or the upper arm, rather than by the axilla. The lever arm is thus shorter than for an axillary crutch, although this is seldom a problem, and they usually run less risk of tissue damage, as well as being lighter and more acceptable cosmetically. In the normal forearm crutch, most of the vertical force is transmitted through the hand but the use of a 'gutter' or 'platform' permits more load to be taken by the forearm itself (Fig. 3.19 right).

Walking frames

The most stable walking aid is the frame, also called a 'walker' or 'Zimmer frame', which enables the subject to stand and walk within the area of support provided by its base. Considerable force can be applied to the frame vertically and moderate forces can be applied horizontally, provided that the overall force vector remains within the area of support. The usual method of walking is first to move the frame forwards, then to take a short step with each foot, then to move the frame again and so on. Walking is thus extremely slow, with a start–stop pattern. Although the subject is encouraged to lift the frame forward at each step, they are more often simply slid along the ground.

A *rollator* is a variant on the walking frame, in which the front feet are replaced by wheels. This makes it easier to advance, at the expense of a slight reduction in stability in the direction of progression. The mode of walking is very similar to that with the frame, except that it is easier to move forwards, since tipping the rollator lifts the back feet clear of the ground. Again, many subjects misuse the rollator by sliding it forwards, rather than tipping it. A further variant on the design is to replace all four feet by wheels, which works well if effective brakes are provided. There are many other designs of frames and rollators, including ones which fold, ones with 'gutters' to support the body weight through the forearms, and ones in which the two sides are connected at the back, rather than at the front.

Gait patterns with walking aids

There are a number of different ways of walking when using a cane, crutch or walker. The terminology varies somewhat from one author to another; the descriptions which follow are based on the well-illustrated text by Pierson (1994). The first four gait patterns involve the greatest support from the upper limbs, by means of a walking frame, two crutches or two canes. The last two require less support, with a crutch or cane held in only one hand.

1. Four-point gait can be employed with canes or crutches. Also known as 'reciprocal gait', it involves the separate and alternate movement of each of the two legs and the two walking aids, for example: left crutch – right leg – right crutch – left leg (Fig. 3.20). This pattern is very stable and requires little energy but it is very slow, so that the oxygen cost (oxygen consumption per unit distance) may be higher than for the three-point gait described below.

2. Three-point gait is used when only one leg can take weight or the two legs move together as a single unit. It is only used with crutches or a walker. Two main forms of three-point gait are recognized: *step-through* and *step-to*. These terms are used when the lower limb musculature is able to provide the movement of the legs. If the legs are paralyzed and their movement is provided by the upper limbs and trunk, the terms *swing-through* and *swing-to* are used (Pierson, 1994). In step-through gait, the foot or feet move from behind the line of the two crutches to in front of them (Fig. 3.21). This gait pattern requires a lot of energy and good control of balance but it can be fairly fast. In step-to gait, the foot or feet are advanced to just behind the line of the crutches, which are then moved further forwards and the process repeated

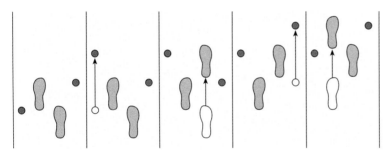

Fig. 3.20 Four-point gait. One crutch or leg is moved at a time in the pattern: left crutch – right leg – right crutch – left leg.

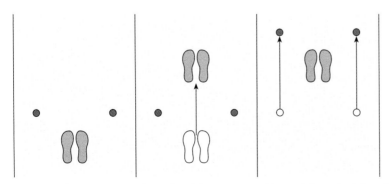

Fig. 3.21 Three-point step-through gait in someone taking weight on both legs. The legs are advanced together, in front of the line of the crutches, then the crutches are advanced together, in front of the line of the legs.

(Fig. 3.22). Since the stride length is short, walking speed is slow but energy and stability requirements are not as high as for step-through gait.

3. Modified three-point gait (also known as *three-one gait*) may be used when one leg is able to take full body weight but the other is not. It may be employed with a walker or with two crutches or canes. The walking aids and the affected leg move forward together, while weight is taken on the sound leg. That leg is then advanced, while weight is taken on the bad leg and the walking aids. This makes for a stable gait pattern, requiring little strength or energy, but the speed is fairly low.

4. Two-point gait resembles four-point gait, except that the crutch or cane on one side is moved forward at the same time as the leg on the other, for example: left crutch/right leg – right crutch/left leg. It is faster than four-point gait, yet is still fairly stable and requires little energy. However, it demands good coordination by the subject.

5. Modified four-point gait is performed when the walking aid is carried in the opposite hand to the affected leg. This gait pattern is typically used in hemiplegia, where there is paralysis of an arm and a leg on the same side. A typical walking sequence would be right crutch – left leg – right leg.

6. Modified two-point gait also involves the use of a walking aid on the opposite side to the bad leg, but the walking aid and the bad leg are moved forward together, for example: right crutch/left leg – right leg. It clearly needs better strength and coordination than modified four-point gait, but gives better speed.

   The stop–start gait pattern seen with some walking aids (especially frames) is known as an 'arrest gait'.

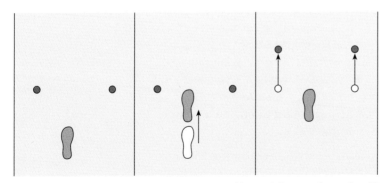

Fig. 3.22 Three-point step-to gait in someone taking weight on only one leg. The leg is advanced to behind the line of the crutches, which are then moved forwards again.

AMPUTEE GAIT

The majority of lower limb amputations are carried out at one of three levels: above knee (AK), below knee (BK) or at the level of the ankle (Syme's). Above knee and below knee amputations are often referred to as *transfemoral* and *transtibial* amputations, respectively. The degree of disability is significantly greater for AK amputees than for the other two groups. As a general rule, amputation at any level is likely to increase the energy expenditure in walking, although how much will depend on the level of amputation, the prosthetic components used and their alignment (Schmalz *et al.*, 2002). Nonetheless, people can adapt remarkably well to amputation, as demonstrated by those individuals who are able to run using an AK prosthesis.

Providing the amputation is carried out competently and the remaining muscles and nerves are normal, people with an AK amputation should have useful function in all the muscle groups acting about the hip joint. However, the mechanical coupling between the femur and the prosthetic limb can never be as good as in the normal individual, for three reasons:

1. The lever arm between the hip joint and the socket is relatively short, which reduces the moment which the hip muscles can apply to the prosthetic leg
2. There is always some relative motion between the stump of the femur and the socket, due to the compression of soft tissues, which is exaggerated in the case of a poorly fitting socket
3. If the socket is uncomfortable, the subject may be reluctant to apply large forces to the prosthetic limb.

AK amputees lack any ability to resist an external flexion moment at the knee and they must walk with the knee in full extension. They commonly use the gait modification of anterior trunk bending in order to keep the knee fully extended. In order to minimize the need for this gait modification, the flexion axis of prosthetic knee joints is normally placed more posteriorly than that of the natural knee, making it easier to keep the force vector in front of the joint. Walking with a stiff knee in the stance phase leads to greater rise and fall of the center of gravity than normal (loss of the third determinant of gait, p. 91) and a consequent increase in energy expenditure. This type of walking is tiring, but nonetheless some people with one or even two AK amputations manage to get around extremely well. There have been some attempts to provide stance phase knee flexion, or its equivalent (shortening the leg through a telescopic action), but these devices have not yet come into widespread use.

Control of the knee joint in the swing phase is one of the most important requirements in the design of an AK prosthesis. If the knee joint is completely free, the pendulum action causes it to flex too quickly following toe off, so that the heel flicks up behind the subject. The knee then extends too rapidly, stopping abruptly as it hits the end stop in hyperextension. In contrast, a knee which permits no flexion or extension requires the whole leg to be accelerated and decelerated in one piece, which places enormous demands on the hip musculature and leads to much higher energy expenditure in walking (Saunders *et al.*, 1953). The compromise between these extremes is a prosthetic knee joint with some form of damping mechanism, which prevents all of these problems.

A variety of different damping mechanisms are available, including friction, hydraulic, pneumatic and computer-controlled systems. Murray *et al.* (1983) examined the gait of AK amputees using two different knee mechanisms, one of which gave a constant frictional load at all knee angles and one, using hydraulics, which varied its loading with knee angle and direction of motion. They found that the performance of the hydraulic mechanism was generally better. Amongst the differences they noted between normal and AK amputee gait, the duration of the swing phase was found to be longer on the amputated side, which resulted in an increased cycle time (decreased cadence). The stride length was close to normal, but the increased cycle time led to a decreased speed. Lateral trunk bending was often present; they attributed this partly to a compensation for a wider walking base, which was used to improve stability, and partly to a compensation for a decreased efficiency of the hip abductors, due to movement of the femoral stump within the socket. Heel rise took place earlier in the stance phase than in normal individuals, because of a reduction in the ability to dorsiflex the prosthetic ankle. The magnitude of the heel rise in initial swing was increased, especially at higher walking speeds; it is very sensitive to the frictional properties of the knee mechanism. There was a tendency to vault on the normal leg during the swing phase of the prosthetic leg. Since the prosthetic leg shortened adequately during the swing phase, this vaulting was probably not necessary. It may have been used to gain added security, since the ground clearance of the prosthetic limb cannot be judged, in the absence of proprioception. Unilateral amputees commonly show other abnormalities in the gait pattern of the sound limb.

Figure 3.23 shows plots of the sagittal plane hip, knee and ankle angles in a 17-year-old female AK amputee with a hydraulic knee mechanism. It should be compared with Fig. 2.5, which shows comparable data from a normal subject. The knee moves into a few degrees of hyperextension well before the end of the swing phase and remains hyperextended until pre-swing. The swing phase knee flexion is almost normal. The stance phase is a little shorter than normal. The hip movement is almost normal, except for a sudden increase in flexion late in the swing phase, as the knee mechanism reaches its extension stop and the momentum of the swinging leg is transferred to the femur. Flexibility in the prosthetic foot leads to a fairly normal pattern of ankle motion, although the magnitudes of these movements are less than normal.

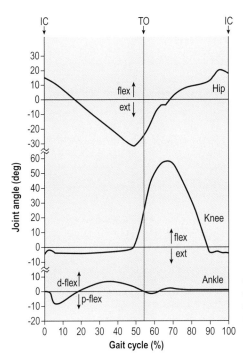

Fig. 3.23 Sagittal plane hip, knee and ankle angles during walking in an above knee amputee. The main abnormality is hyperextension of the knee, from before initial contact to just before toe off. Abbreviations as in Fig. 2.5.

A below knee amputation deprives the user of the ability to plantarflex and dorsiflex the ankle, although the artificial foot normally provides some flexibility in this respect and its shape provides partially functioning initial and terminal rockers. The loss of active plantarflexion at the end of the stance phase means that muscle power cannot be used to provide an active 'push off' and the effective length of the leg is shorter than normal, so that it has to be lifted clear of the ground sooner (Breakey, 1976). According to Saunders *et al.* (1953), the path of the center of gravity is essentially normal after a BK amputation, since the hip and knee together can largely compensate for the loss of the ankle joint. If both ankle and knee are lost, as in an AK amputation, the compensation is incomplete.

Figure 3.24 shows the sagittal plane hip, knee and ankle angles of a 47-year-old male BK amputee using a 'multiflex' foot, walking with a cycle time of 1.26 s (cadence 95 steps/min), stride length 1.45 m and speed 1.15 m/s, all of which are towards the lower end of the normal range. The hip and knee angles are within normal limits. The ankle angle is also nearly normal, although the movement into plantarflexion at the end of the stance phase is of relatively low magnitude and occurs a little late. This is because it is a passive movement, resulting from the removal of loading from the elastic foot mechanism, rather than the active plantarflexion seen in normal subjects.

Figure 3.25 shows the sagittal plane angle, moment and power from the prosthetic ankle of a 35-year-old male BK amputee, using a prosthesis with a SACH foot (solid ankle, cushion heel), walking with a cycle time of 1.13 s (cadence 106 steps/min), stride length 1.54 m and speed 1.37 m/s. The

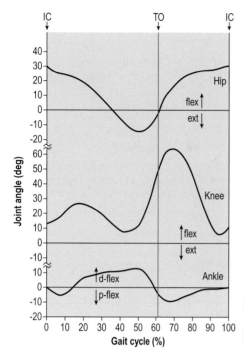

Fig. 3.24 Sagittal plane hip, knee and ankle angles during walking in a below knee amputee. The ankle angle shows slight abnormalities. Abbreviations as in Fig. 2.5.

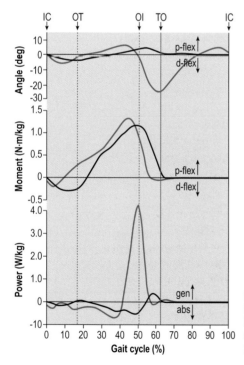

Fig. 3.25 Sagittal plane ankle angle, internal moment and power in a below knee amputee (black line) and normal subject (blue line). Abbreviations as in Figs 2.5–2.7.

corresponding records from the normal subject used for illustration in Chapter 2 are shown as blue lines. The ankle range of motion during the gait cycle in this subject was very restricted, with no plantarflexion around toe off. The ankle moment shows that the prosthesis attempted to retain a fairly neutral position, resisting plantarflexion during the loading response and resisting dorsiflexion during mid-stance and terminal stance. As a result, little power exchange took place until terminal stance, when the ankle absorbed a little power in becoming maximally dorsiflexed. Part of this was returned in power generation as the moment reduced and the ankle returned towards the neutral position. However, the power generation involved was very small, when compared with the normal individual. Other designs of prosthetic foot are better able to store and return energy and research continues in this area.

As can be seen from Figures 3.24 and 3.25, there are considerable differences between subjects in amputee gait. Neither pattern corresponded particularly well to the description by Breakey (1976) of the 'typical' gait pattern of the BK amputee:

1. Delayed foot flat
2. Reduced stance phase knee flexion
3. Early heel rise
4. Early toe off
5. Reduced stance phase duration
6. Reduced swing phase knee flexion.

TREADMILL GAIT

It is often more convenient to study gait while the subject walks on a treadmill rather than over the ground, since the volume in which measurements need to be made is much smaller and they can conveniently be connected to wires or breathing tubes. However, there are subtle differences between treadmill and overground gait, particularly with regard to joint angles. The reduced airflow over the body is unlikely to be a significant factor, but the subject's awareness of the limited length of the treadmill belt may cause them to shorten their stride. However, the most important differences are probably due to changes in the speed of the treadmill belt, as the subject's feet decelerate it at initial contact and accelerate it at push off, effectively storing energy in the treadmill motor. This effect is minimized by using a large treadmill with a powerful motor (Savelberg et al., 1998).

COMMON PATHOLOGIES AFFECTING GAIT

While many pathological conditions can cause an abnormal gait, a group of neurological conditions stand out as being particularly important. If the basic defect is in the brain, the gait abnormality is often very complex and accurate diagnosis may only be possible using the techniques of systematic gait analysis. In contrast, gait abnormalities due to more 'peripheral' disorders, such as diseases of the joints, tend to be much easier to identify and interpret. The following sections outline the gait disorders which may result from some relatively common conditions which affect the brain.

Cerebral palsy

Cerebral palsy is such an important cause of pathological gait, and the main application for clinical gait assessment, that it warrants its own chapter (Chapter 6).

Myelomeningocele

Myelomeningocele (often loosely referred to as 'spina bifida') results from a failure of the lower part of the spinal cord to develop normally. Depending largely on how much of the spinal cord is affected, the neurological deficit may range from negligible to extensive. Many individuals with this condition are able to walk, and gait analysis is often used for assessment and planning treatment (Õunpuu *et al.*, 1996).

Vankoski *et al.* (1995) divided children with the mildest (lumbosacral) form of myelomeningocele into three groups, on the basis of plantarflexor muscle strength, group II being the most affected, group IB being intermediate and group IA the least affected. Group IA patients could generally walk without the use of an ankle–foot orthosis (AFO). The plantarflexor strength generally correlated with the strength of other muscle groups, especially the hip extensors. The authors illustrated the patterns of motion of the pelvis, hip and knee for individuals in all three groups, with and without AFOs.

Parkinsonism

The condition known as parkinsonism (also known as Parkinson's disease) is a disorder of the extrapyramidal system, caused by degeneration of the basal ganglia of the brain. Amongst its other clinical features, it includes a *shuffling gait*. Murray *et al.* (1978) examined the gait of 44 men with parkinsonism and identified the following abnormalities:

1. Stride length and speed were very much reduced, although cycle time (cadence) was usually normal
2. The walking base was slightly increased
3. The range of motion at the hip, knee and ankle were all decreased, mainly by a reduction in joint extension
4. The swinging of the arms was much reduced
5. The majority of patients rotated the trunk in phase with the pelvis, instead of twisting it in the opposite direction
6. The vertical trajectories of the head, heel and toe were all reduced, although other workers have commented on a distinct 'bobbing' motion of the head.

The 'shuffle' occurred because the foot was still moving forward at the time of initial contact. In some patients initial contact was made by the flat foot; in others there was a heelstrike but the foot was much more horizontal than usual. Some patients also showed scuffing of the foot in mid-swing. Unlike most gait patterns, which stabilize within the first two or three steps, the gait of patients with parkinsonism often 'evolves' over the course of several strides.

Other conditions

As was mentioned previously, many different conditions affect gait, only a few of which have been described in detail. Cerebral palsy, myelomeningocele and parkinsonism were singled out for a more detailed discussion, since they can be extremely complicated and often lead to combinations of different gait deviations. The effects of these and other conditions will be further considered in Chapter 5, which deals with the practical application of the methods of gait analysis.

References and suggestions for further reading

Breakey J. (1976) Gait of unilateral below-knee amputees. *Orthotics and Prosthetics* **30**: 17–24.

Gurney B. (2002) Leg length discrepancy. *Gait and Posture* **15**: 195–206.

Lim R, Dias L, Vankoski S *et al.* (1998) Valgus knee stress in lumbosacral myelomeningocele: a gait-analysis evaluation. *Journal of Pediatric Orthopaedics* **18**: 428–433.

Murray MP, Sepic SB, Gardner GM *et al.* (1978) Walking patterns of men with parkinsonism. *American Journal of Physical Medicine* **57**: 278–294.

Murray MP, Mollinger LA, Sepic SB *et al.* (1983) Gait patterns in above-knee amputee patients: hydraulic swing control vs constant-friction knee components. *Archives of Physical Medicine and Rehabilitation* **64**: 339–345.

New York University. (1986) *Lower Limb Orthotics*. New York: New York University Postgraduate Medical School.

Ōunpuu S, Davis RB, DeLuca PA. (1996) Joint kinetics: methods, interpretation and treatment decision-making in children with cerebral palsy and myelomeningocele. *Gait and Posture* **4**: 62–78.

Perry J. (1992) *Gait Analysis: Normal and Pathological Function.* Thorofare, NJ: Slack Incorporated.

Pierson FM. (1994) *Principles and Techniques of Patient Care.* Philadelphia, PA: W.B. Saunders Co.

Saunders JBDM, Inman VT, Eberhart HS. (1953) The major determinants in normal and pathological gait. *Journal of Bone and Joint Surgery* **35**: 543–558.

Savelberg HHCM, Vorstenbosch MATM, Kamman EH *et al.* (1998) Intra-stride belt-speed variation affects treadmill locomotion. *Gait and Posture* **7**: 26–34.

Schmalz T, Blumentritt S, Jarasch R. (2002) Energy expenditure and biomechanical characteristics of lower limb amputee gait: the influence of prosthetic alignment and different prosthetic components. *Gait and Posture* **16**: 255–263.

Vankoski SJ, Sarwark JF, Moore C *et al.* (1995) Characteristic pelvic, hip and knee kinematic patterns in children with lumbosacral myelomeningocele. *Gait and Posture* **3**: 51–57.

Methods of gait analysis

4

Gait analysis is used for two very different purposes: to aid directly in the treatment of individual patients and to improve our understanding of gait, through research. Gait research use may be further subdivided into 'fundamental' studies of walking and clinical research. These topics are explored further in the next chapter. Clearly, no single method of analysis is suitable for such a wide range of uses and a number of different methodologies have been developed.

When considering the methods which may be used to perform gait analysis, it is helpful to regard them as being in a 'spectrum' or 'continuum', ranging from the absence of technological aids, at one extreme, to the use of complicated and expensive equipment at the other. This chapter starts with a method which requires no equipment at all and goes on to describe progressively more elaborate systems. As a general rule, the more elaborate the system, the higher the cost, but the better the quality of objective data that can be provided. However, this does not imply that some of the simpler techniques are not worth using. It has often been found, particularly in a clinical setting, that the use of high-technology gait analysis is inappropriate, because of its high cost in terms of money, space and time, and because the clinical problem can be adequately managed using simpler techniques.

VISUAL GAIT ANALYSIS

It is tempting to say that the simplest form of gait analysis is that made by the unaided human eye. This, of course, neglects the remarkable abilities of the human brain to process the data received by the eye. Visual gait analysis is, in reality, the most complicated and versatile form of analysis available. Despite this, it suffers from four serious limitations:

1. It is transitory, giving no permanent record
2. The eye cannot observe high-speed events
3. It is only possible to observe movements, not forces
4. It depends entirely on the skill of the individual observer.

In a study on the reproducibility of visual gait analysis, Krebs *et al.* (1985) found it to be 'only moderately reliable'. Saleh & Murdoch (1985) compared the performance of people skilled in visual gait analysis with the data provided by a combined kinetic/kinematic system. They found that the measurement system identified many more gait abnormalities than had been seen by the observers.

Many clinicians include the observation of a subject's gait as part of their clinical examination. However, this is not gait analysis if it is limited to watching the subject make a single walk, up and down the room. This merely gives a superficial idea of how well they walk and perhaps identifies the most serious abnormality. A thorough visual gait analysis, as recommended in the manual from New York University (1986), involves watching the subject while he or she makes a number of walks, some of which are observed from one side, some from the other side, some from the front and some from the back. As the subject walks, the observer should look for the presence or absence of a number of specific gait abnormalities, such as those described in Chapter 3 and summarized in Table 4.1. A logical order should be used for looking for the

Table 4.1 Common gait abnormalities and best direction for observation

Gait abnormality	Observing direction
Lateral trunk bending	Side
Anterior trunk bending	Side
Posterior trunk bending	Side
Increased lumbar lordosis	Side
Circumduction	Front or behind
Hip hiking	Front or behind
Steppage	Side
Vaulting	Side or front
Abnormal hip rotation	Front or behind
Excessive knee extension	Side
Excessive knee flexion	Side
Inadequate dorsiflexion control	Side
Abnormal foot contact	Front or behind
Abnormal foot rotation	Front or behind
Insufficient push off	Side
Abnormal walking base	Front or behind
Rhythmic disturbances	Side

different gait abnormalities – the mixture of walking directions listed in the table is not recommended! According to Rose (1983), it is also important, when performing visual gait analysis, to compare the ranges of motion at the joints during walking with those which are observed on the examination plinth – they may be either greater or smaller.

The minimum length required for a gait analysis walkway is a hotly debated subject. The author believes that 8 m (26 ft) is about the minimum for use with fit young people, but that 10–12 m (33–39 ft) is preferable, since it permits fast walkers to 'get into their stride' before any measurements are made. However, shorter walkways are satisfactory for people who walk more slowly. This particularly applies to those with a pathological gait, since the gait pattern usually stabilizes within the first two or three steps. A notable exception to this, however, is the gait in parkinsonism, which 'evolves' over the first few strides. The width required for a walkway depends on what equipment, if any, is being used to make measurements. For visual gait analysis, as little as 3 m (10 ft) may be sufficient. If video recording is being used, the camera needs to be positioned a little further from the subject and about 4 m (13 ft) is needed. A kinematic system making simultaneous measurements from both sides of the body normally requires a width of at least 5–6 m (16–20 ft). Figure 4.1 shows the layout of a small gait laboratory used for visual gait analysis, video recording and the measurement of the general gait parameters.

Some investigators permit subjects to choose their own walking speed, whereas others control the cycle time (or cadence), for example by asking them to walk in time with a metronome. The rationale for controlling the cycle time is that many of the measurable parameters of gait vary with the walking speed and using a controlled cycle time provides one means of reducing the variability. However, subjects are unlikely to walk naturally when trying to keep pace with a metronome, and patients with motor control problems may find it difficult or even impossible to walk at an imposed cycle

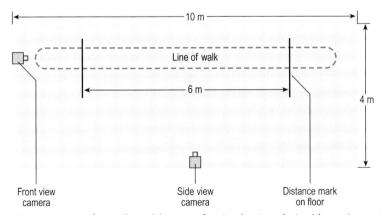

Fig. 4.1 Layout of a small gait laboratory for visual gait analysis, videotaping and measurement of the general gait parameters.

time. Zijlstra *et al.* (1995) found considerable differences in the gait of normal subjects between 'natural' walking and 'constrained' walking, in which the subject was required either to step in time with a metronome or to step on particular places on the ground. The answer to this dilemma is probably to accept the fact that subjects need to walk at different speeds and to interpret the data appropriately. This means that 'normal' values must be available for a range of walking speeds. An unresolved difficulty with this approach is that it may not be possible to get 'normal' values for very slow walking speeds, since normal individuals do not customarily walk very slowly and when asked to do so, some of the gait measurements become very variable (Brandstater *et al.*, 1983).

Gait assessment

Simply observing the gait and noting abnormalities is of little value by itself. It needs to be followed by gait assessment, which is the synthesis of these observations with other information about the subject, obtained from the history and physical examination, combined with the intelligence and experience of the observer (Rose, 1983). Visual gait analysis is entirely subjective and the quality of the analysis depends on the skill of the person performing it. It can be an interesting exercise to perform visual gait analysis on people walking past in the street, but without knowing their clinical details it is easy to misinterpret what is wrong with them.

When performing any type of gait analysis, one thing that must be constantly borne in mind is that you are observing effects and not causes. Putting it another way, the observed gait pattern is not the direct result of a pathological process but the net result of a pathological process and the subject's attempts to compensate for it. The observed gait pattern is 'what is left after the available mechanisms for compensation have been exhausted' (Rose, 1983).

Examination by video recording

The widespread use of videotape and direct recording to a digital versatile disk (DVD) or computer has provided one of the most useful enhancements to gait analysis during recent years. It helps to overcome two of the limitations of visual gait analysis: the lack of a permanent record and the difficulty of observing high-speed events. In addition, it confers the following advantages:

1. It reduces the number of walks a subject needs to do
2. It makes it possible to show the subject exactly how they are walking
3. It makes it easier to teach visual gait analysis to someone else.

Gait examination by video recording is not an objective method, since it does not provide quantitative data in the form of numbers. However, it does provide a permanent record, which can be extremely valuable. The presence of an earlier recording of a subject's gait may be used to demonstrate to all concerned how much progress has been made, especially when this has occurred over a long period of time. In particular, it may convince a subject or family member that an improvement *has* occurred, when memory tells them that they are no better than they were several months ago!

When using videotape, the most practical system consists of a camera-recorder ('camcorder'), to do the videotaping and a separate video cassette recorder (VCR) to replay the tapes. The majority of today's domestic camcorders are perfectly suitable for use in gait analysis, the requirements being a zoom lens, automatic focus, the ability to operate in normal room lighting and an electronically shuttered charge-coupled device (CCD) sensor, to eliminate blurring due to movement. The VCR used to view the tapes should have a rock-steady freeze-frame facility, without any 'stripes' across the picture, and the ability to single-step successive frames, either one at a time or at a very slow speed. Such features are now available on many domestic VCRs, making them perfectly suitable for use in a clinical gait laboratory. Videotape may thus be used to visualize events which are too fast for the unaided eye. For convenience, the camcorder should use the same size cassette as the VCR which will be used to view the tapes, thus avoiding the need for tape copying. Many gait laboratories now record video data directly into a computer and this may be synchronized with data collection on a kinematic system (described later).

In making a thorough visual gait analysis without the use of video recording, the subject needs to make repeated walks to confirm or refute the presence of each of the gait abnormalities listed in Table 4.1. If the subject is in pain or easily fatigued, this may be an unreasonable requirement and it may be difficult to achieve a satisfactory analysis. The use of video recording permits the subject to do a much smaller number of walks, as the person performing the analysis can watch the recording as many times as necessary.

Video recording facilitates the process of teaching visual gait analysis, in which the student often needs to see small abnormal movements which happen very quickly. It is much easier to see such movements if the gait can be examined in slow motion, with the instructor pointing out details on the television or computer monitor. The use of video recording also makes it possible to observe a variety of abnormal gaits which have been archived. A number of teaching video recordings are now available (Appendix 3).

Showing the subject a video recording of their own gait is not exactly 'biofeedback', since there is a time delay involved, but nonetheless it can be very helpful. When a therapist is working with a subject to correct a gait abnormality, the subject may gain a clearer idea of exactly what the therapist is concerned about if they can observe their own gait from the 'outside'.

Although visual gait analysis using video recording is subjective, it is easy, at the same time, to derive some objective data. The general gait parameters (cycle time or cadence, stride length and speed) can be measured by a method which will be described in the next section (p. 145). It is also possible to measure joint angles, either directly from the monitor screen or using some form of on-screen digitizer. Such measurements tend to be fairly inaccurate, however, because the limb may not be viewed from the correct angle and because of distortions introduced by the television camera, the recording medium and (especially) the television or computer display.

Individual investigators will find their own ways of performing gait analysis using video recording, but the author's own routine may prove useful as a starting point. Subjects are asked to wear shorts or a swim suit, so that the majority of the leg is visible. It is important that the subject should walk as 'normally' as possible, so they are asked to wear their own indoor or outdoor shoes, with socks if preferred. Unless it would unduly tire the subject, it is a good idea to make one or two 'practice' walks, before starting video recording. The camera position, or the zoom lens, is first adjusted to show the whole body from head to feet and the subject is recorded from the side, as they walk the length of the walkway in one direction. At the end, they turn around, with a rest if necessary, and are recorded as they walk back again. The whole process is then repeated, with the camera adjusted to show a close-up of the body from the waist down. Then either the camera position is changed or the subject is asked to walk along a different pathway, so that they can be recorded while walking away from the camera and then back towards it again. Two walks in each direction are again recorded, although the magnification does not need to be changed, since this view automatically provides a range of views from close-up to full-body.

It is often helpful to mark the subject's skin, for example using an eyebrow pencil, to enhance the visibility of anatomical landmarks on the recording. Hillman *et al.* (1998) fitted subjects with surface-mounted 'rotation indicators', to improve the accuracy with which transverse plane rotations can be estimated from video recording.

Subjects should not be able to see themselves on a monitor while they are walking, as this provides a distraction, particularly for children. Whether they are shown the video recording afterwards is at the discretion of the investigator, although it is important to review the recording before the subject leaves, in case it needs to be repeated for some reason.

The analysis is performed by replaying the video recording, looking for specific gait abnormalities in the different views and interpreting what is seen in the light of the subject's history and physical examination. It is particularly helpful if two or more people work together to perform the analysis. Rose (1983) suggested that gait analysis should be based on the team approach, with discussion and hypothesis testing. As will be described in Chapter 5, hypothesis testing may involve an attempted modification of the gait, for instance by fitting an orthosis or by paralyzing a muscle using local anesthetic.

GENERAL GAIT PARAMETERS

The general gait parameters (also known as the temporal and distance factors of gait) are the cycle time (or cadence), stride length and speed. These provide the simplest form of objective gait evaluation (Robinson & Smidt, 1981). Although there are automatic ways of making these measurements, which will be described in the next section, they may also be made using only a stopwatch, a tape measure and (optionally) some talcum powder. The method described below, under 'general gait parameters from video recording', enables the simultaneous measurement of all three of the general gait parameters and does not actually require the patient's gait to be recorded, since it can be used while the patient's gait is being observed.

Cycle time, stride length and speed tend to change together in most locomotor disabilities, so that a subject with a long cycle time will usually also have a short stride length and a low speed (speed being stride length divided by cycle time). The general gait parameters give a guide to the walking ability of a subject, but little specific information. They should always be interpreted in terms of the expected values for the subject's age and sex, such as those given in Appendix 1. Figure 4.2 shows one way in which these data may be presented; the diamonds represent the 95% confidence limits for a normal subject of the same age and sex as the subject under investigation. Although cycle time is gradually replacing cadence in the gait analysis community, it is more convenient to use cadence on plots of this type, since abnormally slow gait will give values on the left-hand side of the graph for all three of the general gait parameters.

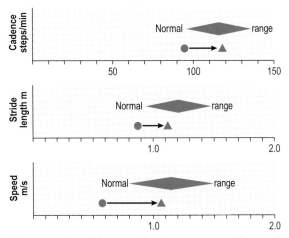

Fig. 4.2 Display of the general gait parameters, with normal ranges appropriate for a patient's age and sex. Pre- and postoperative values for a 70-year-old female patient undergoing knee replacement surgery.

Cycle time or cadence may be measured with the aid of a stopwatch, by counting the number of individual steps taken during a known period of time. It is seldom practical to count for a full minute, so a period of 10 or 15 seconds is usually chosen. The loss of accuracy incurred by counting for such short periods of time is unlikely to be of any practical significance. The subject should be told to walk naturally and they should be allowed to get up to their full walking speed before the observer starts to count the steps. The cycle time is calculated using the formula:

cycle time (s) = time (s) × 2/steps counted

The number '2' allows for the fact that there are two steps per stride. The cadence is calculated using the formula:

cadence (steps/min) = steps counted × 60/time (s)

The number '60' allows for the fact that there are 60 seconds in a minute.

Stride length

Stride length can be determined in two ways: by direct measurement or indirectly from the speed and cycle time. The simplest direct method of measurement is to count the strides taken while the subject covers a known distance. A more useful method (but a rather messy one!) is to have the subject step with both feet in a shallow tray of talcum powder and then walk across a polished floor or along a strip of brown wrapping paper or colored 'construction paper', leaving a trail of footprints. These may be measured, as shown in Fig. 2.3, to derive left and right step lengths, stride length, walking base, toe out angle and some idea of the foot contact pattern. This investigation is able to provide a great deal of useful information, for the sake of a few minutes of mopping up the floor afterwards! As an alternative to using talcum powder, felt adhesive pads, soaked in different colored dyes, may be fixed to the feet (Rose, 1983). The subject walks along a strip of paper and leaves a pattern of dots, which give an accurate indication of the locations of both feet.

If both the cycle time and the speed have been measured, stride length may be calculated using the formula:

stride length (m) = speed (m/s) × cycle time (s)

The equivalent calculation using cadence is:

stride length (m) = speed (m/s) × 2 × 60/cadence (steps/min)

The multiplication by '2' converts steps to strides and by '60' converts minutes to seconds. For accurate results, the cycle time and speed should be measured during the same walk. However, the simultaneous counting, measuring and timing may prove too difficult and the errors introduced by using data from different walks are not likely to be important, unless the subject's gait varies markedly from one walk to another.

Speed

The speed may be measured by timing the subject while he or she walks a known distance, for example between two marks on the floor or between two pillars in a corridor. The distance walked is a matter of convenience but somewhere in the region of 6–10 m (20–33 ft) is probably adequate. Again, the subject should be told to walk at their natural speed and they should be allowed to get into their stride before the measurement starts. The speed is calculated as follows:

speed (m/s) = distance (m)/time (s)

General gait parameters from video recording

Determination of the general gait parameters from a video recording of the subject walking is easy, providing the recording shows the subject passing two landmarks whose positions are known. One simple method is have the subject walk across two lines on the floor, a known distance apart, made with adhesive tape. Space should be allowed for acceleration before the first line and for slowing down after the second one. When the recording is replayed, the time taken to cover the distance is measured and the steps taken are counted. It is easiest to take the first initial contact *beyond the start line* as the point to begin both timing and counting and the first initial contact *beyond the finish line* as the point to end both timing and counting. The first step beyond the start line must be counted as 'zero', not 'one'. This method of measurement is not strictly accurate, since the position of the foot at initial contact is an unknown distance beyond the start and finish line, but the errors introduced are unlikely to be significant. As mentioned above, this method can also be employed without the use of video recording.

Since the distance, the time and the number of steps are all known, the general gait parameters can be calculated using the formulae:

cycle time (s) = time (s) × 2/steps counted
cadence (steps/min) = steps counted × 60/time (s)
stride length (m) = distance (m) × 2/steps counted
speed (m/s) = distance (m)/time (s)

TIMING THE GAIT CYCLE

A number of systems have been described which perform the automatic measurement of the timing of the gait cycle, sometimes called the temporal gait parameters. Such systems may be divided into two main classes: footswitches and instrumented walkways. Figure 4.3 shows typical data, which could be obtained from either type of system.

Footswitches

Footswitches are used to record the timing of gait. If one switch is fixed beneath the heel and one beneath the forefoot, it is possible to measure the timing of initial contact, foot flat, heel rise and toe off, and the duration of the stance phase (see Figs 2.2 and 4.3). Data from two or more strides make it

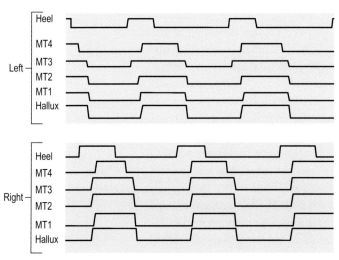

Fig. 4.3 Output from footswitches under the heel, four metatarsals (MT 1 to MT 4) and hallux of both feet. The switch is 'on' (i.e. the area is in contact with the ground) when the line is high.

possible to calculate cycle time and swing phase duration. If switches are mounted on both feet, the single and double support times can also be measured. The footswitches are usually connected through a trailing wire to a computer, although alternatively either a radio transmitter or a portable recording device may be used to collect the data and transfer them to the measuring equipment.

A footswitch is exposed to very high forces, which may cause problems with reliability. This has led to many different designs being tried over the years. A fairly reliable footswitch may be made from two layers of metal mesh, separated by a thin sheet of plastic foam with a hole in it. When pressure is applied, the sheets of mesh contact each other through the hole and complete an electrical circuit. Footswitches are most conveniently used with shoes, although suitably designed ones may be taped directly beneath the foot. Small switches may also be mounted in an insole and worn inside the shoe. In addition to the basic heel and forefoot switches, further switches may be used in other areas of the foot, to give greater detail on the temporal patterns of loading and unloading. In addition to the home-made varieties, a number of companies also manufacture footswitches.

Instrumented walkways

An instrumented walkway is used to measure the timing of foot contact, the position of the foot on the ground, or both. Many different designs have been developed, usually individually built for a single laboratory. The descriptions which follow refer to typical designs, rather than to any particular system.

A conductive walkway is a gait analysis walkway which is covered with an electrically conductive substance, such as sheet metal, metal mesh or conductive rubber. Suitably positioned electrical contacts on the subject's shoes complete an electrical circuit. The conductive walkway is thus a slightly different method of implementing footswitches and provides essentially the same information. Again, the subject usually trails an electrical cable, which connects the foot contacts to a computer. The speed needs to be determined independently, typically by having the body of the subject interrupt the beams of two photoelectric cells, one at each end of the walkway, again connected to the computer. Timing information from the foot contacts is used to calculate the cycle time, and the combination of cycle time and speed may be used to calculate the stride length.

An alternative arrangement is to have the walkway itself contain a large number of switch contacts, which detect the position of the foot, as well as the timing of heel contact and toe off. This has the advantage that no trailing wires are required and the walkway can be used to measure both step lengths and the stride length. A number of commercial systems are available to make this type of measurement, often also providing some information on the magnitude of the forces between the foot and the ground. One such system, which is now in common use, is the 'GAITRite' (Bilney *et al.*, 2003; Menz *et al.*, 2004).

DIRECT MOTION MEASUREMENT SYSTEMS

A number of systems have been described which measure the motion of the body or legs, using some form of direct connection to the subject. As a general rule, direct measurement systems are more likely to be found in research laboratories than in clinical settings and they are gradually giving way to other methods of measurement.

The simplest of these systems measures the forward displacement of the trunk, by means of a light string, which is connected to the back of a belt around the subject's waist. As the individual walks forwards, the string is pulled through an instrument which measures its motion. This may be achieved in a number of ways, including a tacho-generator, which is a form of dynamo, the output voltage of which relates to the instantaneous speed of the string, or a device such as an optical encoder, which can be used to measure the length of the string as it passes through. Such systems will give the mean speed of walking and also the instantaneous speed as it changes during the gait cycle.

A more elaborate system, based on the same principle, may be used to measure pelvic twist about the vertical axis, by having one string attached to each side of the waist. It is also possible to measure lateral displacement in walking, by having one or two strings running sideways, although some means must be provided to cope with the forward motion, such as by having the subject walk on a treadmill.

Direct connection systems may also be used to measure the motion of the legs. One such system uses perforated paper tape, attached to the heels of both shoes, which is pulled through an optical reader as the subject walks forwards (Law, 1987; Law & Minns, 1989). This gives timing and displacement information for both feet, enabling the calculation of the cycle time, the two step lengths, stride length, speed, stance and swing phase durations and the two double support times. Another system which gives similar information is based on a small trolley which is towed along behind the subject by a loop of cord, the ends of which are attached to the two feet (Klenerman *et al.*, 1988). The cord runs backwards and forwards through a measuring instrument on the trolley and its movements provide the temporal and distance parameters of gait. The designers of both systems claimed that the subject is not aware of any drag produced by the attachments to the feet.

ELECTROGONIOMETERS

An electrogoniometer is a device for making continuous measurements of the angle of a joint. The output of an electrogoniometer is usually plotted as a chart of joint angle against time, as shown in Fig. 2.5. However, if measurements have been made from two joints (typically the hip and the knee), the data may be plotted as an *angle-angle diagram*, also known as a 'cyclogram', shown in Fig. 4.4. This format makes clearer the interaction between the two joints and makes it possible to identify characteristic patterns.

Potentiometer devices

A rotary potentiometer is a variable resistor of the type used as a radio volume control, in which turning the central spindle produces a change in electrical resistance, which can be measured by an external circuit. It can be used to measure the angle of a joint if it is fixed in such a way that the body of the potentiometer is attached to one limb segment and the spindle to the other. The electrical output thus depends on the joint position and the device can be calibrated to measure the joint angle in degrees. Many laboratories have constructed their own electrogoniometers of this type and there have in the past been a few commercially available designs.

Although any joint motion could be measured by an electrogoniometer, they are most commonly used for the knee and less commonly for the ankle and hip. Fixation is usually achieved by cuffs, which wrap around the limb segment above and below the joint. The position of the potentiometer is adjusted to be as close to the joint axis as possible. A single potentiometer will only make measurements in one axis of the joint, but two or three may be mounted in different planes to make multiaxial measurements (Fig. 4.5).

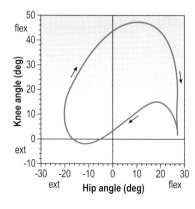

Fig. 4.4 Angle-angle diagram of the sagittal plane hip angle (horizontal axis) and knee angle (vertical axis). Initial contact is at the lower right. Normal subject; same data as Fig. 2.6.

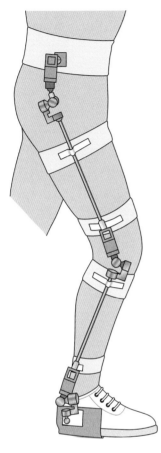

Fig. 4.5 Subject wearing triaxial goniometers on hip, knee and ankle. Adapted from manufacturer's literature (Chattecx Corporation).

Trailing wires are normally used to connect the potentiometers to the measuring equipment, which is usually a computer.

Concern has been expressed about the accuracy of measurement provided by these potentiometer devices, since they are subject to a number of possible types of error, described below.

1. The electrogoniometer is fixed by cuffs around the soft tissues, not to the bones, so that the output of the potentiometer does not exactly relate to the true bone-on-bone movement at the joint.
2. Some designs of electrogoniometer will only give a true measurement of joint motion if the potentiometer axis is aligned to the anatomical axis of the joint. This may not be achievable for three reasons:
   • it may be difficult to identify the joint axis, e.g. because of the depth of the hip joint below the surface
   • the joint axis may not be fixed, e.g. the 'polycentric' flexion–extension axis of the knee
   • the rotation axis may be inaccessible, e.g. the internal–external rotation axis of the knee.

3. A joint may, in theory, move with up to six degrees of freedom – that is, it may have angular motion about three mutually perpendicular axes and linear motion ('translations') in three directions. In practice, the linear motion is usually negligible, particularly at the hip and ankle, and most electrogoniometer systems simply 'lose' any motion which does occur, either through the elasticity of the mounting cuffs or through a sliding or 'parallelogram' mechanical linkage. However, where the electrogoniometer axis does not correspond exactly with the anatomical axis, larger linear motions will occur.

4. The output of the device gives a relative angle rather than an absolute one and it may be difficult to decide what limb angle should be taken as 'zero', particularly in the presence of a fixed deformity.

Because of these problems, electrogoniometers are more popular in a clinical setting, in which great accuracy is not usually needed, than in the scientific laboratory. Chao (1980) addressed some of these problems, in a defense of the use of potentiometer-based electrogoniometers in gait analysis.

Flexible strain gauges

The flexible strain gauge electrogoniometer (Fig. 4.6), manufactured by Biometrics Ltd (Cwmfelinfach, Gwent, UK), consists of a flat, thin strip of metal, one end of which is fixed to the limb on each side of the joint being studied. The bending of the metal as the joint moves is measured by strain gauges and their associated electronics. Because of the way in which metal strips respond to bending, the output depends simply on the angle between the two ends, linear motion being ignored. To measure motion in more than one axis, a two-axis goniometer may be used, or two or three separate goniometers may be fixed around the joint, aligned to different planes.

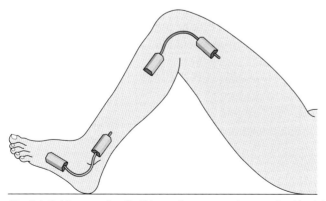

Fig. 4.6 Subject wearing flexible goniometers on knee and ankle. Adapted from manufacturer's literature (Biometrics Ltd).

Other electrogoniometers

With the increasing use of television-based kinematic systems (see below), electrogoniometers are declining in popularity. Other designs which have been used in the past include mercury-in-rubber, in which the electrical resistance of a column of mercury in an elastic tube changes as the tube is stretched across a joint, and an optical system known as the polarized light goniometer.

PRESSURE BENEATH THE FOOT

The measurement of the pressure beneath the foot is a specialized form of gait analysis, which may be of particular value in conditions in which the pressure may be excessive, such as diabetic neuropathy and rheumatoid arthritis. Lord *et al.* (1986) reviewed a number of such systems. Foot pressure measurement systems may be either floor mounted or in the form of an insole within the shoe.

The SI unit for pressure is the pascal (Pa), which is a pressure of one newton per square meter. The pascal is inconveniently small, and practical measurements are made in kilopascals (kPa) or megapascals (MPa). Conversions between different units of measurement will be found in Appendix 2.

Lord *et al.* (1986) pointed out that when making measurements beneath the feet, it is important to distinguish between force and pressure (force per unit area). Some of the measurement systems measure the force (or 'load') over a known area, from which the mean pressure over that area can be calculated. However, the mean pressure may be much lower than the peak pressure within the area if high pressure gradients are present, which are often caused by subcutaneous bony prominences, such as the metatarsal heads.

A pitfall which must be borne in mind when making pressure measurements beneath the feet is that a subject will normally avoid walking on a painful area. Thus, an area of the foot which had previously experienced a high pressure and has become painful may show a low pressure when it is tested. However, this will not happen if the sole of the foot is anesthetic, as commonly occurs in diabetic neuropathy. In this condition, very high pressures, leading to ulceration, may be recorded.

Typical pressures beneath the foot are 80–100 kPa in standing, 200–500 kPa in walking and up to 1500 kPa in some sporting activities. In diabetic neuropathy, pressures as high as 1000–3000 kPa have been recorded. To put these figures into perspective, the normal systolic blood pressure, measured at the feet in the standing position, is below 33 kPa (250 mmHg); applied pressures which are higher than this will prevent blood from reaching the tissues.

Glass plate examination

Some useful semi-quantitative information on the pressure beneath the foot can be obtained by having the subject stand on, or walk across, a glass plate, which is viewed from below with the aid of a mirror or television camera. It is easy to see which areas of the sole of the foot come into contact with the walking surface and the blanching of the skin gives an idea of the applied pressure. Inspection of both the inside and the outside of a subject's shoe will also provide useful information about the way the foot is used in walking; it is a good idea to ask patients to wear their oldest shoes when they come for an examination, not their newest ones!

Direct pressure mapping systems

A number of low-technology methods of estimating pressure beneath the foot have been described over the years. The Harris or Harris–Beath mat is made of thin rubber, the upper surface of which consists of a pattern of ridges of different heights. Before use, it is coated with printing ink and covered by a sheet of paper, after which the subject is asked to walk across it. The highest ridges compress under relatively light pressures, the lower ones requiring progressively greater pressures, making the transfer of ink to the paper greater in the areas of the highest pressure. This gives a semi-quantitative map of the pressure distribution beneath the foot. Other systems have also been described, in which the subject walks on a pressure-sensitive film, a sheet of aluminum foil or on something like a typist's carbon paper.

Pedobarograph

The Pedobarograph uses an elastic mat, laid on top of an edge-lit glass plate. When the subject walks on the mat it is compressed onto the glass, which loses its reflectivity, becoming progressively darker with increasing pressure. This darkening provides the means for quantitative measurement. The underside of the glass plate is usually viewed by a television camera, the monochrome image being processed to give a 'false-color' display, in which different colors correspond to different levels of pressure.

Force sensor systems

A number of systems have been described in which the subject walks across an array of force sensors, each of which measures the vertical force beneath a particular area of the foot. Dividing the force by the area of the cell gives the mean pressure beneath the foot in that area. Many different types of force sensor have been used, including resistive and capacitative strain gauges, conductive rubber, piezoelectric materials and a photoelastic optical system. A number of different methods have been used to display the output of such systems, including the attractive presentation shown in Fig. 4.7.

In-shoe devices

The problem of measuring the pressure inside the shoe has been tackled in a number of centers. The main difficulties with this type of measurement are the curvature of the surface, a lack of space for the transducers and the need to run large numbers of wires from inside the shoe to the measuring equipment. Nonetheless, a number of commercial systems are now available, which may give clinically useful results. Details of such systems may be found on the Internet (Appendix 3).

ELECTROMYOGRAPHY

Electromyography (EMG) is the measurement of the electrical activity of a contracting muscle – the muscle action potential. Since it is a measure of

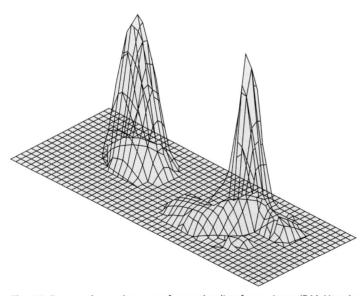

Fig. 4.7 Pressure beneath a cavus foot on landing from a jump (E.M. Hennig, 5th Biennial Conference, Canadian Society of Biomechanics, 1988).

electrical and not mechanical activity, the EMG cannot be used to distinguish between concentric, isometric and eccentric contractions, and the relationship between EMG activity and the force of contraction is far from straightforward. One of the most useful textbooks on the EMG is that by Basmajian (1974). The use of the EMG in the biomechanical analysis of movement was reviewed by Kleissen *et al.* (1998).

The three methods of recording the EMG are by means of surface, fine wire and needle electrodes. In gait analysis, EMG is usually measured with the subject walking, as opposed to the semi-static EMG measurements which are often made for neurological diagnosis.

Surface electrodes

Surface electrodes are fixed to the skin over the muscle, the EMG being recorded as the voltage difference between two electrodes. It is usually necessary also to have a grounding electrode, either nearby or elsewhere on the body. Since the muscle action potential reaches the electrodes through the intervening layers of fascia, fat and skin, the voltage of the signal is relatively small and it is usually amplified close to the electrodes, using a very small pre-amplifier. The EMG signal picked up by surface electrodes is the sum of the muscle action potentials from many motor units within the most superficial muscle or muscles. Most of the signal comes from within 25 mm of the skin surface, so this type of recording is not suitable for deep muscles such as the iliopsoas. The EMG data may not be very specific, even with superficial muscles, due to interference from adjacent muscles ('cross-talk'). It is safest to regard the signal from surface electrodes as being derived from muscle groups, rather than from individual muscles, although Õunpuu *et al.* (1997) showed that surface electrodes could satisfactorily distinguish between the three superficial muscle bellies of the quadriceps in children. There is often a change in the electrical baseline as the subject moves ('movement artifact') and there may also be electromagnetic interference, for example from nearby electrical equipment.

Fine wire electrodes

Fine wire electrodes are introduced directly into a muscle, using a hypodermic needle which is then withdrawn, leaving the wires in place. They can be quite uncomfortable or even painful. The wire is insulated, except for a few millimeters at the tip. The EMG signal may be recorded in three different ways:

1. Between a pair of wires inserted using a single needle
2. Between two fine wires, inserted separately
3. Between a single fine wire and a ground electrode.

The voltage recorded within the muscle is generally higher than that from surface electrodes, particularly if separate wires are used, and there is less interference from movement and from electromagnetic fields. The signal is derived from a fairly small region of a single muscle, generally from a few motor units, a fact which must be taken into account when interpreting the data. Because it is an uncomfortable and invasive technique, fine wire EMG is usually only performed on selected muscles, in patients in whom it is likely to be particularly useful.

Needle electrodes

Needle electrodes are generally more appropriate to physiological research than to gait analysis. A hypodermic needle is used, which contains an insulated central conductor. This records the EMG signal from a very local area within the muscle into which it is inserted, usually only a single motor unit.

Limitations of EMG

The main problem with the use of any form of EMG is that it is at best only a semi-quantitative technique and gives little indication of the strength of contraction of individual muscles. Many attempts have been made over the years to make it more quantitative, with only limited success. The other problem with EMG is that it may be quite difficult to obtain satisfactory recordings from a walking subject. This depends partly on the electronic characteristics of the equipment being used and partly on the skill of the operator in selecting the recording sites and in attaching the electrodes, to minimize skin resistance and movement artifacts. The EMG signal is generally processed to provide a visible indication of muscle activity.

Despite its limitations, the information provided by EMG on the timing of muscle activation can be of considerable value in gait assessment. For example, one form of treatment in cerebral palsy is to transfer the tendon of a muscle to a different position, thereby altering the action of the muscle. When contemplating this type of surgery, it is essential to use EMG first, to make sure that the timing of muscular contraction is appropriate for its new role.

ENERGY CONSUMPTION

The most accurate way of measuring the total amount of energy used in performing an activity such as walking is 'whole-body calorimetry', in which the subject is kept in an insulated chamber, from which the heat output of the body can be measured. This is, of course, quite impractical, except as a research technique. The most usual way of estimating energy expenditure is based on measuring the body's oxygen consumption. There are also less direct methods, using either mechanical calculations or the measurement of heart rate.

Oxygen consumption

The measurement of oxygen consumption requires an analysis of the subject's exhaled breath. If both the volume of exhaled air and its oxygen content are measured, the amount of oxygen consumed in a given time can be calculated. The amount of carbon dioxide produced can also be measured and the ratio of the carbon dioxide produced to the oxygen consumed (the 'respiratory quotient') provides information on the type of metabolism which is taking place (aerobic or anaerobic). Except under abnormal environmental conditions, it is not necessary to measure either the oxygen or the carbon dioxide in the inspired air, since these are almost constant.

The classic method of measuring oxygen consumption and carbon dioxide production is to fit the subject with a noseclip and mouthpiece and to collect the whole of the expired air in a large plastic or rubberized canvas 'Douglas bag' or a meteorological balloon. If the subject is walking, some means of following them around with the bag is needed. A small sample of the gas in the bag is then analyzed, after which the volume of exhalate in the bag is measured. After correcting for temperature, air pressure and humidity, a very accurate estimate of oxygen consumption can be obtained. However, collecting the expirate in this way is uncomfortable for the subject and the technique is quite unsuitable for some patients. A less cumbersome, though potentially slightly less accurate method again involves a noseclip and mouthpiece, but uses a portable system which performs continuous gas sampling and volume measurement, so that it is not necessary to collect the whole of the expirate. Either form of gas collection can be achieved using a facemask, rather than a mouthpiece and noseclip, although it may be very difficult either to prevent leakage or to detect leakage if it does occur. The use of a portable system with a facemask is routine in some gait analysis centers, who find that even children accept it well. Occasionally, studies of locomotion are made using a spirometer, in which the subject breathes in and out of an oxygen-filled closed system, which absorbs the exhaled carbon dioxide. Since spirometers are not usually portable, they are practical only when walking on a treadmill.

Mechanical calculations

It was pointed out in Chapter 1 (p. 43) that the expenditure of metabolic energy does not result in the production of an equivalent amount of mechanical work. Indeed, in eccentric muscular activity, metabolic energy is used to absorb, rather than to generate, mechanical energy. Even when muscular contraction is used to do positive work, the efficiency of conversion is relatively low, as well as being variable and difficult to estimate. For these reasons, it is generally unsatisfactory to use mechanical calculations to estimate the total metabolic energy consumed in a complicated activity such as walking. Nonetheless, this method of estimating energy expenditure is used in some laboratories (Gage *et al.*, 1984) and is known as the 'estimated external work of walking' (EEWW). Calculations of this type are more reliable for activities where the relationship between the muscular contraction and the mechanical output is extremely simple, such as in the concentric contraction of a single muscle.

Even though mechanical calculations are generally unsatisfactory for the estimation of the total energy consumption of the body, the measurement of the energy generation and transfer at individual joints may be of great value in gait analysis. Results of such measurements were given in Chapters 2 and 3. They may be made using combined kinetic/kinematic systems, which are described at the end of this chapter.

Heart rate monitoring

Rose (1983) stated that heart rate monitoring is a good substitute for the measurement of oxygen uptake, since a number of studies over the years have shown that there is a surprisingly close relationship between the two. Heart rate monitoring is certainly much easier to perform and there are a number of systems available, often based on detecting the pulsatile flow in the capillaries, for example in the finger. Another method of recording heart rate is to detect the electrocardiogram, using electrodes mounted on the chest. As a general rule, the energy consumption is related to the difference in heart rate between the resting condition and that measured during the exercise. Rather than attempting to relate the change in heart rate directly to energy consumption, some investigators use the 'physiological cost index' (PCI), which is said to be less sensitive to differences between individuals (Steven *et al.*, 1983). It is calculated as follows:

PCI = (heart rate walking − heart rate resting)/speed

The calculation must be made using consistent units, with the heart rate in beats per minute and the speed in meters per minute, or the heart rate in beats per second and the speed in meters per second. The measurement unit for the PCI is net beats per meter. Since the heart rate tends to be somewhat variable, small changes in PCI may not be significant.

ACCELEROMETERS

Accelerometers, as their name suggests, measure acceleration. Typically, they contain a small mass, connected to a stiff spring, with some electrical means of measuring the spring deflection when the mass is accelerated. The type of accelerometer used in gait analysis is usually very small, weighing only a few grams. It normally only measures acceleration in one direction, but more than one may be grouped together for two- or three-dimensional measurements. Solid-state accelerometers, built as integrated circuits, are also available. Because of their small size, they may be of value in gait analysis and also in providing feedback for future systems involving powered artificial limbs and orthoses.

Typically, accelerometers have been used for gait analysis in one of two ways: either to measure transient events or to measure the motion of the limbs.

Measurement of transients

Accelerometers are very suitable for measuring brief, high-acceleration events, such as the heelstrike transient. Johnson (1990) described the development of an accelerometer system to assess the performance of shock-attenuating footwear, which was made available commercially.

The main difficulty with this type of measurement is in obtaining an adequate mechanical linkage between the accelerometer and the skeleton, since slippage occurs in both the skin and the subcutaneous tissues. On a few occasions, experiments have been performed with accelerometers mounted on pins, screwed directly into the bones of volunteers. Reviews of this subject were published by Collins & Whittle (1989) and Whittle (1999).

The use of accelerometers for the kinematic analysis of limb motion has been explored by a number of research workers, notably Morris (1973). If the acceleration of a limb segment is known, a single mathematical integration will give its velocity and a second integration its position, providing both position and velocity are known at some point during the measurement period. However, these requirements, combined with the 'drift' from which accelerometers often suffer, have prevented them from coming into widespread use for this purpose. If the limb rotates as well as changing its position, which is usually the case, further accelerometers are needed to measure the angular acceleration.

Trunk accelerations have been used to measure the general gait parameters (Zijlstra & Hof, 2003). This is an extension of the principle behind the 'pedometer', often carried by hikers, which counts steps by measuring the vertical accelerations of the trunk.

GYROSCOPES

It has been suggested that gyroscopes could be used to measure the orientation of the body segments in space and that 'rate-gyros' could be used to measure angular velocity and acceleration. Gyroscopes have been used on an experimental basis in some gait laboratories and the development of very small solid-state devices may make this a useful method of measurement in the future. Nene *et al.* (1999) used a gyroscope, in combination with several accelerometers, in a study of thigh and shank motion during the swing phase of gait.

FORCE PLATFORMS

The force platform, which is also known as a 'forceplate', is used to measure the ground reaction force as a subject walks across it (Fig. 4.8). Although many specialized types of force platform have been developed over the years, most clinical laboratories use a commercial platform, a 'typical' design being about 100 mm high, with a flat rectangular upper surface measuring 400 mm by 600 mm. To make the upper surface extremely rigid, it is either made of a large piece of metal or of a lightweight honeycomb structure. Within the platform, a number of transducers are used to measure tiny displacements of the upper surface, in all three axes, when force is applied to it. The electrical output of the platform may be provided as either eight channels or six. An eight channel output consists of:

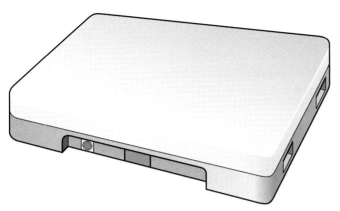

Fig. 4.8 Force platform. Adapted from manufacturer's literature (AMTI Inc.).

1. Four vertical signals, from transducers near the corners of the platform
2. Two fore–aft signals from the sides of the platform
3. Two side-to-side signals, from the front and back of the platform.

A six channel output generally consists of:

1. Three force vector magnitudes
2. Three moments of force, in a coordinate system based on the center of the platform.

Although it is possible to use the output signal from a force platform directly, for example by displaying it on an oscilloscope, it is much more usual to collect it into a computer, through an analog-to-digital converter. Neither the eight channel nor the six channel force platform output is particularly convenient for biomechanical calculations and it is usual to convert the data to some other form. Regrettably, no standard has been established for the coordinate systems used for either kinetic or kinematic data.

Ideally, a force platform should be mounted below floor level, the upper surface being flush with the floor. If this is not possible, it is usual to build a slightly raised walkway, to accommodate the thickness of the platform. It is highly undesirable to have the subject step up onto the platform and then down off it again, since such a step could never be regarded as 'normal' walking. Force platforms are very sensitive to building vibrations and many early gait laboratories were built in basements, to reduce this form of interference. In the author's opinion, this problem has been overemphasized, since although building vibrations can be seen in force platform data, they are negligible when compared with the magnitude of the signals recorded from subjects walking on the platform.

One problem which may be experienced when using force platforms is that of 'aiming'. To obtain good data, the whole of the subject's foot must land on the platform. It is tempting to tell the subject where the platform is and to ask them to make sure that their footstep lands squarely on it. However, this is likely to lead to an artificial gait pattern, as the subject 'aims' for the platform. If at all possible, the platform should be disguised so that it is not noticeably different from the rest of the floor and the subject should not be informed of its presence. This may require a number of walks to be made, with slight adjustments in the starting position, before acceptable data can be obtained.

Where it is required to record from both feet, the relative positioning of two force platforms can be a considerable problem. There is no single arrangement which is satisfactory for all subjects, and some laboratories have designed systems in which one or both platforms can be moved, to suit the gait of individual subjects. Figure 4.9 shows the arrangement used in a number of laboratories, which is a reasonable compromise for studies on adults but is unsatisfactory when the stride length is either very short or very long. For subjects who have a very short stride length, such as children, better results may be obtained if the platforms are mounted with their shorter dimensions in the direction of the walk. Alternatively, the direction of the walk may be altered, to cross the platforms diagonally. Despite these strategies, the problem may be insoluble. For example, Gage *et al.* (1984) observed that 'force plate data were discounted because the smaller children frequently stepped on the same platform twice because of their short stride lengths'. Some laboratories improve their chances of obtaining good data by using three or four force platforms.

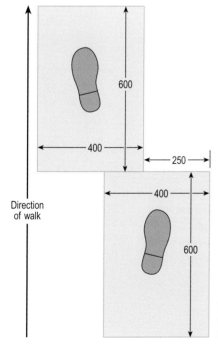

Direction of walk

Fig. 4.9 Typical arrangement of two force platforms for use in studies of adults (dimensions in mm).

It is often impossible to get the whole of one foot on one force platform and the whole of the other foot on the other one, without also having unwanted additional steps on one or other platform. To some extent, computer software can be used to 'unscramble' the data when both feet have stepped on one platform but, more commonly, it is necessary to use the data from only one foot at a time.

The usual methods of displaying force platform data are:

1. Individual components, plotted against time (see Fig. 2.19)
2. The 'butterfly diagram' (see Fig. 2.8)
3. The center of pressure (see Figs 2.20 and 2.21).

In the latter case, if it is required to superimpose a foot outline in the correct position on the plot, it is necessary also to measure the position of the foot on the force platform, for example by using talcum powder.

A number of things have to be borne in mind when interpreting force platform data. Firstly, although the foot is the only part of the body in contact with the platform, the forces which are transmitted by the foot are derived from the mass and inertia of the whole body. The force platform has been described as a 'whole-body accelerometer'; its output gives the acceleration in three-dimensional space of the center of gravity of the body as a whole, including both the limb which is on the ground and the leg which is swinging through the air. This means that changes in total body inertia may swamp small changes in ground reaction force due to events occurring within the foot. For example, fairly high moments are recorded about the vertical axis during the stance phase of gait (Fig. 4.10). While these may be slightly

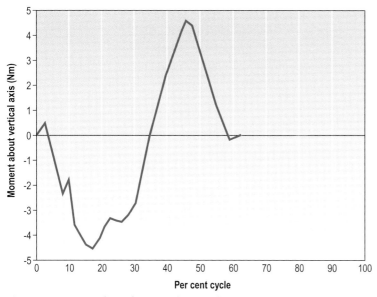

Fig. 4.10 Moments about the vertical axis at the instantaneous center of pressure, during the stance phase of gait. Normal subject, right leg. A positive moment occurs when the foot attempts to move clockwise relative to the floor.

modified by local events within the foot, they are mainly derived from the acceleration and retardation of the other leg, as it goes through the swing phase. The reaction to the forces responsible for this acceleration and retardation are transmitted to the floor through the stance phase leg and appear in the force platform output, principally as a torque about the vertical axis.

When interpreting force platform data, it is also helpful to remember that force is equivalent to the rate of change of momentum. If two objects of identical mass are dropped onto a force platform from the same height, one which bounces will produce a higher ground reaction force than one which does not. This may at first seem surprising, until it is realized that the change in momentum is twice as much for the object which bounces as it is for the one which does not.

It can be difficult to measure transients, such as the heelstrike, with a force platform. This is because the top plate is usually fairly massive and does not respond well to very brief forces. The heelstrike transient shown in Fig. 2.22 was recorded using a newer design (Bertec), with a stiff but lightweight top plate, giving it a high frequency response. When measuring transients, it is important not to pass the data through a low pass filter. If the data are sampled using a computer analog-to-digital converter, the sampling rate needs to be high enough to record the waveform accurately (1000 Hz in Fig. 2.22).

Force platform data by themselves are of limited value in gait analysis. Nevertheless, some laboratories use them empirically, for example by looking for particular patterns in the 'butterfly diagram' (Rose, 1985) or comparing the heights of the different peaks and troughs. Some inferences can also be made from the shapes of the curves of the individual force components. For example, there is an association between stance phase flexion of the knee and a dip at mid-stance in the vertical component of force. However, the true value of the force platform is only appreciated when the ground reaction force data are combined with kinematic data. The combination provides a much more complete mechanical description of gait than either by itself and permits the calculation of joint moments and powers.

A number of workers have developed devices which are not force platforms but have the same function. Typically, they consist of a small number of force sensors, which are fixed to the sole of a shoe. As the subject walks, the electrical output gives the ground reaction force and the center of pressure. Typically only the vertical component of the ground reaction force is measured, although at least one three-axis system has been described. The advantages claimed are:

1. The ability to measure multiple steps
2. No problems with 'aiming'
3. No risk of stepping on the platform with both feet
4. No risk of or missing the platform, either partly or completely.

The disadvantages are the presence of the force sensors beneath the feet, and the associated wiring. Also, the coordinate system for the force measurements moves with the foot, in contrast to the room-based coordinate system used for kinematic data. This makes it very difficult to combine the two types of data, to perform a full biomechanical analysis.

Force platforms may also be used for balance testing and the measurement of postural sway, which are important in some forms of neurological diagnosis. For a complete analysis of the balance mechanism, however, it is necessary to provide some means whereby both the supporting surface and the visual environment may be moved relative to the subject.

KINEMATIC SYSTEMS

Kinematics is the measurement of movement or, more specifically, the geometric description of motion, in terms of displacements, velocities and accelerations. Kinematic systems are used in gait analysis to record the position and orientation of the body segments, the angles of the joints and the corresponding linear and angular velocities and accelerations.

Following the pioneering work of Marey and Muybridge in the 1870s, photography remained the method of choice for the measurement of human movement for about 100 years, until it was replaced by electronic systems. Two basic photographic techniques were used: *cine photography* and *multiple-exposure photography*. Cine photography is achieved by the use of a series of separate photographs, taken in quick succession. Multiple exposure photography has existed in many different forms over the years. It is based on the use of a single photograph, or a strip of film on which a series of images are superimposed, sometimes with a horizontal displacement between each image and the next. The 1960s and 1970s saw the development of gait analysis systems based on *optoelectronic techniques*, including television, and these have now superseded photographic methods.

The general principles of kinematic measurement are common to all systems and will be discussed before considering particular systems in detail.

General principles

Kinematic measurement may be made in either two dimensions or three. Three-dimensional measurements normally require the use of two or more cameras, although methods have been devised in which a single camera can be used to make limited three-dimensional measurements.

The simplest kinematic measurements are made using a single camera, in an uncalibrated system. Such measurements are fairly inaccurate but they may be useful for some purposes. Without calibration, it is impossible to measure distances accurately and such a system is normally used only to measure joint angles in the sagittal plane. The camera is positioned at right angles to the plane of motion and as far away as possible, to minimize the distortions introduced by perspective. To give a reasonable size image, with a long camera-to-subject distance, a 'telephoto' (long focal length) lens is used. The angles measured from the image are projections of three-dimensional angles onto a two-dimensional plane and any part of the angulation which occurs out of that plane is ignored. Commercial systems of this type are available for measuring joint angles from television images. Such measurements may be subject to yet another form of error, since the horizontal and vertical scales of a television image may be different.

A single-camera system can be used to make approximate measurements of distance, if some form of calibration object is used, such as a grid of known dimensions behind the subject. Measurement accuracy will be lost by any movement towards or away from the camera, but this effect can again be minimized if the camera is a long distance away from the subject, using a telephoto lens. Angulations of the limb segments, either towards or away from the camera, will also interfere with length measurements.

To achieve reasonable accuracy in kinematic measurement, it is necessary to use a calibrated three-dimensional system, which involves making measurements from more than one viewpoint. A detailed review of the technical aspects of the three-dimensional measurement of human movement was given in four companion papers by Capozzo *et al.* (2005), Chiari *et al.* (2005), Leardini *et al.* (2005) and Della Croce *et al.* (2005). Although there are considerable differences in convenience and accuracy between cine film, videotape, television/computer and optoelectronic systems, the data processing for the different types of three-dimensional measurement systems is similar.

Most commercial kinematic systems use a three-dimensional calibration object, which is viewed by all the cameras, either simultaneously or in sequence. Computer software is used to calculate the relationship between the known three-dimensional positions of 'markers' on the calibration object and the two-dimensional positions of those markers in the fields of view of the different cameras. An alternative method of calibration is used by the Coda system, whose optoelectronic sensors are in fixed relation to each other, permitting the system to be calibrated in the factory.

When a subject walks in front of the cameras, the calibration process is reversed and three-dimensional positions are calculated for the markers fixed to the subject's limbs, so long as they are visible to at least two cameras. Data are collected at a series of time intervals known as 'frames'. Most systems have an interval between frames of either 20 ms, 16.7 ms or 5 ms, corresponding to data collection frequencies of 50 Hz, 60 Hz or 200 Hz, although some systems now offer frame rates beyond 200 Hz. When a marker can be seen by only one camera, its three-dimensional position cannot be calculated, although it may be estimated by 'interpolation', using data from earlier and later frames.

All measurement systems, including the kinematic systems to be described, suffer from measurement errors. Measurement accuracy depends to a large extent on the field of view of the cameras, although it also differs somewhat between the different systems. The earlier systems had measurement errors of 2–3 mm in all three dimensions, throughout a volume large enough to cover a complete gait cycle (Whittle, 1982). Recently, design and (especially) calibration improvements have reduced typical errors to less than 1 mm. Some commercial systems claim to provide much higher accuracy than this, but the author treats such claims with skepticism, particularly when applied to the measurement of moving markers under realistic gait laboratory conditions.

Technical descriptions of kinematic systems use, and sometimes misuse, the terms 'resolution', 'precision' and 'accuracy'. In practical terms, *resolution* means the ability of the system to measure small changes in marker position. *Precision* is a measure of system 'noise', being based on the amount of variability there is between one frame of data and the next. For the majority of users, the most important parameter is *accuracy*, which describes the relationship between where the markers really are and where the system says they are!

Most commercial systems are sufficiently accurate to measure the positions of the limbs and the angles of the joints. However, the calculation of linear or angular velocity requires the mathematical differentiation of the position data, which magnifies any measurement errors. A second differentiation is required to determine acceleration, and a small amount of measurement 'noise' in the original data leads to wildly erratic and often unusable results for acceleration. The usual way of avoiding this problem is to smooth the position data, using a low-pass filter, before differentiation. This achieves the desired object but means that any genuinely high accelerations, such as that at the heelstrike transient, are lost.

Thus, kinematic systems are good at measuring position but poor at determining acceleration, because of the problems of differentiating even slightly noisy data. Conversely, accelerometers are good at measuring acceleration but poor at estimating position, because of the problems of integrating data with baseline drift. Really accurate data could be obtained by combining the two methods, using each to correct the other and calculating the velocity from both. Some research studies have been conducted using this combined approach.

As well as the errors inherent in measuring the positions of the markers, further errors are introduced because considerable movement may take place between a skin marker and the underlying bone. A few studies have been performed (e.g. Holden *et al.*, 1997; Reinschmidt *et al.*, 1997) in which steel pins were inserted into the bones of 'volunteers' (usually the investigators themselves) and the positions of skin markers compared with the positions of markers on the pins. The amount of skin movement revealed by such studies is generally somewhat worrying! The amount of error this causes in the final result depends on which parameter is being measured. For example, marker movement has little effect on the sagittal plane knee angle, because it causes only a small relative change in the length of fairly long segments, but it may cause considerable errors in transverse plane measurements or on measurements involving shorter segments, such as in the foot. In some cases, the magnitude of the error is greater than the measurement itself! Skin movement may also introduce significant errors in the calculation of joint moments and powers. A possibility for the future is to correct for marker movement, by estimating the movement relative to the underlying bone.

A further error is introduced when the positions of the joints are estimated from anthropometric measures (e.g. leg length) and the positions of skin markers, particularly where it is possible to place the markers in the wrong position. Even for subjects with normal anatomy, these errors can be substantial; for patients with bony deformity, the errors may be even greater. This is a field in which improvements continue to be made.

There are two fundamentally different approaches to positioning markers on the limbs. One method is to mount each marker directly on the skin, generally over a bony anatomical landmark. The position and orientation of the limb segment are then defined by the marker positions, and the position of the joint center is calculated from these locations. The other approach is to fix a set of at least three markers to each limb segment, either directly or mounted on a rigid structure (sometimes called a 'pod'), so that its position and orientation can be determined in three-dimensional space. The movement of one limb segment relative to the next, and the position of the joint center, may then be derived mathematically. The joint center may be determined either by 'pointing' to it in a static calibration or by measuring the movements of the pods as the joint moves through its range of motion. Both methods have advantages and disadvantages and both suffer from errors due to marker movement. Rigid plates, in particular, may be moved by the contraction of the underlying muscles. Also, because they are relatively heavy, their inertia causes them to lag behind the limb segment during rapid accelerations. Figure 4.11 shows two possible ways of arranging lower limb markers, one utilizing 'pods' on the thigh and shank and one based on markers mounted over anatomical landmarks.

Mention has already been made of the use of force platforms for the measurement of postural sway. Kinematic systems may also be used to make this type of measurement in the standing individual.

Photographic systems

The author does not know of any laboratories which still use multiple-exposure photography, but a few still use cine. The major disadvantages of using cine film are the cost of the materials, the time taken to process the film

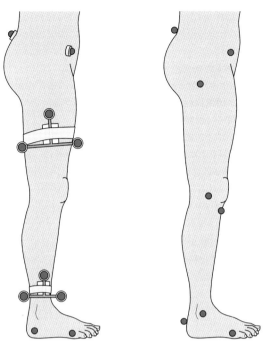

Fig. 4.11 Typical marker configurations for the pelvis and lower limb. Left: using rigid arrays (Cleveland Clinic). Right: skin mounted, over anatomical landmarks (University of Oxford).

and the effort involved in manually digitizing the data. Its advantages are the relatively low cost of the equipment, the potentially high accuracy obtainable and the ability to film subjects 'in the field', rather than in the laboratory. For this last reason, cine photography is still fairly popular for measuring sporting activities, although it is being replaced by video recording. Normal cine cameras expose at speeds of up to 25 frames per second, but special high-speed cameras are usually needed for gait analysis and particularly for sporting activities, to avoid blurring of the image and the loss of detail in movements.

The subject is filmed, using one or more cameras, as he or she performs the activity, whether it be walking or performing some sporting event. If a calibration object is being used, this is also filmed, without altering the camera positions or settings. After the film or films have been processed, the images are digitized by an operator, who views successive frames, identifies the required landmarks and measures their two-dimensional coordinates. Although this can be done using a ruler, graph paper or a microscope with a travelling stage, it is most conveniently performed by projecting the film image onto the surface of a 'digitizing tablet', using a specially designed 'analyzing projector'. The operator moves a cursor to the appropriate points in the image and presses a button to transfer the coordinates of each point into a computer. To avoid inaccuracies caused by frame-to-frame variations in film position, it is common also to digitize the positions of fixed markers within the field of view.

Videotape and DVD digitizers

The use of videotape or DVD to augment visual gait analysis has already been described. Video recording may also be used as the basis for a kinematic system, in the same way that cine photography has been used. It has considerable advantages in terms of cost, convenience and speed, although it may not be quite as accurate, because of the poorer resolution of a television image compared with cine film and the further losses involved in recording and replaying the images. Another considerable advantage, however, is that it is possible to automate the digitization process using electronic processing of the image, especially if skin markers are used, which show up clearly against the background. A number of commercial systems are available, which can be used either as a two-dimensional system with a single camera, or as a three-dimensional system using two or more cameras. Most video recording systems use conventional television equipment, although high-speed systems are also available.

Television/computer systems

A number of different television/computer systems have been developed since 1967. Although the systems differ in detail, the following description is typical.

Reflective markers are fixed to the subject's limbs, either close to the joint centers or fixed to limb segments in such a way as to identify their positions and orientations (Fig. 4.11). Close to the lens of each television camera is an infrared or visible light source, which causes the markers to show up as very bright spots. The markers are usually covered in 'Scotchlite', the material that makes road signs show up brightly when illuminated by car headlights. To avoid the 'smearing' which occurs if the marker is moving, only a short exposure time is used. This may be achieved by one or more of the following:

1. Using stroboscopic illumination
2. Using a mechanical shutter on the camera
3. Using a charge-coupled device (CCD) television camera, which is only enabled (i.e. activated) for a short interval during each frame.

If two or more cameras are used, much more accurate measurements can be made if they are synchronized. For normal purposes, frame rates of 50 Hz, 60 Hz or 200 Hz are used, but specialized systems running at higher speeds are also available. As a general rule, the twin penalties for having the extra speed are increased system cost and a reduction in measurement accuracy.

Each television camera is connected to a special interface board which analyzes each television frame. The systems differ in how they locate the 'centroid' or geometric center of each marker within the television image, but it is typically calculated using the edges of any bright spots in the field of view (Fig. 4.12). Because a large number of edges are used to calculate the position of the centroid, its position can be determined to a greater accuracy than the horizontal and vertical resolution of the television image. This is known as making measurements with 'subpixel accuracy'. Marker centroids may also be calculated using the optical density of all the pixels in the image, rather than just marker edges, again with an improvement in accuracy.

The computer stores the marker centroids from each frame of data for each camera, but initially there is no way to associate a particular marker centroid with a particular physical marker, such as that on the right knee. The process of identifying which marker image is which for each of the cameras, and of following the markers from one frame of data to the next, is known as 'tracking' or 'trajectory following'. The speed and convenience of this process differ considerably from one system to another and also between software options from a single manufacturer. In the past this has been the least satisfactory aspect of television/computer systems, although software improvements have now made it much more straightforward. The main differences between systems are in whether the tracking process has to be undertaken separately for each camera or whether a three-dimensional reconstruction of the data is made before the operator is asked to identify which marker is which. The end result of the tracking and 3-D reconstruction process is a computer file of three-dimensional marker positions.

These systems were originally developed to measure the motion of the lower limbs, but they may also be used to measure motion of the lumbar spine (Whittle & Levine, 1997), the trunk (Crosbie et al., 1997) and the upper limbs. Beyond their use in gait analysis, they are increasingly used to provide the input for computer graphic systems, in the video game and motion picture industries.

A number of television/computer systems are also available which were intended for other purposes, such as aircraft tracking, but which could possibly be adapted for use in gait analysis. Typically, such systems are based

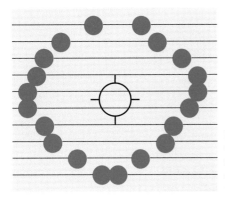

Fig. 4.12 Location of marker centroid (open circle in center) from the position on successive television lines of the leading and trailing edges of the marker image (solid circles).

on the identification of particular shapes in the video image, and they hold the promise of 'markerless' tracking.

Active marker systems

Another type of kinematic system uses active markers, typically light-emitting diodes (LEDs), and a special optoelectronic camera. Typically, these systems use invisible infra-red radiation, but for the sake of clarity, the word 'light' will be used in the following explanation. The camera measures the position of the marker by analyzing the light coming from it, using either two-dimensional or one-dimensional cameras.

The LEDs are arranged to flash on and off in sequence, so that only one is illuminated at any instant of time. The cameras are thus able to locate each marker in turn, without the need for a 'tracking' procedure to determine which one is which. The penalty for this convenience is the need for the subject to carry a power supply, with wires running to each of the markers. Problems may also occur because the camera records not just the light from the LEDs, but any other light which falls on it. This may include stray ambient light, which is fairly easy to eliminate, but also reflections caused by the markers themselves, which in some systems are difficult both to detect and to eliminate. These problems have led to a decline in the popularity of active marker systems, although they are usually very accurate, have a high sampling rate, and are convenient to use.

Other kinematic systems

A number of other methods of making kinematic measurements are in use in different laboratories. Several systems are available which detect, by means of magnetic fields, the position and orientation of small coils of wire, fixed to a subject's limbs. For example, Pearcy & Hindle (1989) developed a method for measuring motion of the lumbar spine, by mounting a source (transmitter) on the sacrum and a sensor (receiver) over the first lumbar vertebra. Systems are also available in which the location of ultrasound transmitters, placed on the subject, is detected by an array of microphones.

COMBINED KINETIC/KINEMATIC SYSTEMS

When a kinematic system, such as one of those described above, is combined with a force platform (which is a kinetic system), the capability of the combined system is greater than that of the sum of its component parts. The reason for this is that if the relationship is known between the limb segments and the ground reaction force vector, it is possible to perform 'inverse dynamic' calculations, in which the limb is treated as a mechanical system. While not all commercial systems provide the necessary software to make these calculations, there exists the potential to calculate the moments of force and the power generated or absorbed at all the major joints of the lower limb. Such calculations require a knowledge of the masses and moments of inertia of the limb segments and the location of their centers of gravity. Direct measurements of these are clearly impossible, but published data, modified to suit the subject's anthropometry, give an acceptable approximation. It is common practice in such calculations to regard the foot as a single rigid object, although this simplification undoubtedly causes errors in calculating the ankle power.

A fully equipped clinical gait laboratory can be expected to possess, as a minimum, a combined kinetic/kinematic system, with ambulatory EMG (Fig. 4.13), as well as facilities for making videotapes (or their equivalent). Equipment may also be available for measuring oxygen uptake or pressure beneath the feet. If the laboratory is also used for research, then further facilities and equipment may also be present.

One of the big problems with kinetic/kinematic systems is that they provide such a wealth of data that it may be very difficult to distinguish between those observations which are important and those which are not. Recent research has used a number of mathematical, statistical and computational techniques

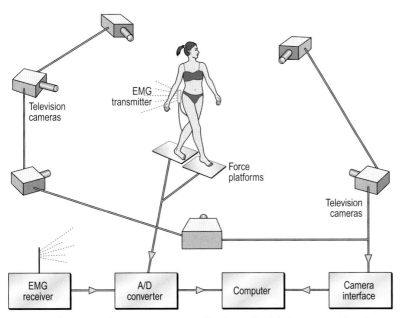

Fig. 4.13 The gait analysis equipment used in the author's laboratory, with a six camera kinematic system, two force platforms and an EMG telemetry system.

in an attempt to address this problem (Chau, 2001a, b), some examples being multivariate analysis, principal component analysis, neural networks and the charmingly named 'fuzzy systems'. It may be anticipated that in the future 'expert systems' will be available to draw the attention of clinicians to those aspects of a patient's gait most in need of attention. Another way of coping with this huge quantity of data is to reduce many different measurements to a single index. An example of this is the 'Normalcy Index' suggested by Schutte *et al.* (2000) as a method of quantifying a patient's disability and providing an outcome measure to gauge their response to treatment, which Romei *et al.* (2004) found to be 'clinically applicable, reliable and easy to use'.

References and suggestions for further reading

Basmajian JV. (1974) *Muscles Alive: Their Functions Revealed by Electromyography.* Baltimore, MD: Williams & Wilkins.

Bilney B, Morris M, Webster K. (2003) Concurrent related validity of the GAITRite walkway system for quantification of the spatial and temporal parameters of gait. *Gait and Posture* **17**: 68–74.

Brandstater ME, de Bruin H, Gowland C *et al.* (1983) Hemiplegic gait: analysis of temporal variables. *Archives of Physical Medicine and Rehabilitation* **64**:583–587.

Capozzo A, Della Croce U, Leardini A *et al.* (2005) Human movement analysis using stereophotogrammetry. Part 1: Theoretical background. *Gait and Posture* **21**: 186–196.

Chao EYS. (1980) Justification of triaxial goniometer for the measurement of joint rotation. *Journal of Biomechanics* **13**:989–1006.

Chau T. (2001a) A review of analytical techniques for gait data. Part 1: fuzzy, statistical and fractal methods. *Gait and Posture* **13**:49–66.

Chau T. (2001b) A review of analytical techniques for gait data. Part 2: neural network and wavelet methods. *Gait and Posture* **13**:102–120.

Chiari L, Della Croce U, Leardini A, *et al.* (2005) Human movement analysis using stereophotogrammetry. Part 2: Instrumental errors. *Gait and Posture* **21**: 197–211.

Collins JJ, Whittle MW. (1989) Impulsive forces during walking and their clinical implications. *Clinical Biomechanics* **4**:179–187.

Crosbie J, Vachalathiti R, Smith R. (1997) Patterns of spinal motion during walking. *Gait and Posture* **5**:6–12.

Della Croce U, Leardini A, Chiari L *et al.* (2005) Human movement analysis using stereophotogrammetry. Part 4: Assessment of anatomical landmark misplacement and its effects on joint kinematics. *Gait and Posture* **21**: 226–237.

Gage JR, Fabian D, Hicks R *et al.* (1984) Pre- and postoperative gait analysis in patients with spastic diplegia: a preliminary report. *Journal of Pediatric Orthopedics* **4**:715–725.

Hillman SJ, Hazlewood ME, Loudon IR *et al.* (1998) Can transverse plane rotations be estimated from video tape gait analysis? *Gait and Posture* **8**:87–90.

Holden JP, Orsini JA, Siegel KL *et al.* (1997) Surface movement errors in shank kinematics and knee kinetics during gait. *Gait and Posture* **5**:217–227.

Johnson GR. (1990) Measurement of shock acceleration during walking and running using the shock meter. *Clinical Biomechanics* **5**:47–50.

Kleissen RFM, Buurke JH, Harlaar J *et al.* (1998) Electromyography in the biomechanical analysis of human movement and its clinical application. *Gait and Posture* **8**:143–158.

Klenerman L, Dobbs RJ, Weller C *et al.* (1988) Bringing gait analysis out of the laboratory and into the clinic. *Age and Ageing* **17**:397–400.

Krebs DE, Edelstein JE, Fishman S. (1985) Reliability of observational kinematic gait analysis. *Physical Therapy* **65**:1027–1033.

Law HT. (1987) Microcomputer-based, low cost method for measurement of spatial and temporal parameters of gait. *Journal of Biomedical Engineering* **9**:115–120.

Law HT, Minns RA. (1989) Measurement of the spatial and temporal parameters of gait. *Physiotherapy* **75**:81–84.

Leardini A, Chiari L, Della Croce U *et al.* (2005) Human movement analysis using stereophotogrammetry. Part 3: Soft tissue artifact assessment and compensation. *Gait and Posture* **21**: 212–225.

Lord M, Reynolds DP, Hughes JR. (1986) Foot pressure measurement: a review of clinical findings. *Journal of Biomedical Engineering* **8**:283–294.

Menz HB, Latt MD, Tiedemann A *et al.* (2004) Reliability of the GAITRite walkway system for the quantification of temporo-spatial parameters of gait in young and older people. *Gait and Posture* **20**: 20–25.

Morris JRW. (1973) Accelerometry – a technique for the measurement of human body movements. *Journal of Biomechanics* **6**:729–736.

Nene A, Mayagoitia R, Veltink P. (1999) Assessment of rectus femoris function during initial swing phase. *Gait and Posture* **9**:1–9.

New York University. (1986) *Lower Limb Orthotics*. New York: New York University Postgraduate Medical School.

Õunpuu S, DeLuca PA, Bell KJ *et al.* (1997) Using surface electrodes for the evaluation of the rectus femoris, vastus medialis and vastus lateralis in children with cerebral palsy. *Gait and Posture* **5**:211–216.

Pearcy MJ, Hindle RJ. (1989) New methods for the non-invasive three-dimensional measurement of human back movement. *Clinical Biomechanics* **4**:73–79.

Reinschmidt C, van den Bogert AJ, Lundberg A *et al.* (1997) Tibiofemoral and tibiocalcaneal motion during walking: external vs. skeletal markers. *Gait and Posture* **6**:98–109.

Robinson JL, Smidt GL. (1981) Quantitative gait evaluation in the clinic. *Physical Therapy* **61**:351–353.

Romei M, Galli M, Motta F *et al.* (2004) Use of the normalcy index for the evaluation of gait pathology. *Gait and Posture* **19**: 85–90.

Rose GK. (1983) Clinical gait assessment: a personal view. *Journal of Medical Engineering and Technology* **7**:273–279.

Rose GK. (1985) Use of ORLAU-Pedotti diagrams in clinical gait assessment. In: Whittle M, Harris D (eds) *Biomechanical Measurement in Orthopaedic Practice*. Oxford: Clarendon Press, pp. 205–210.

Saleh M, Murdoch G. (1985) In defence of gait analysis. *Journal of Bone and Joint Surgery* **67B**:237–241.

Schutte LM, Narayanan U, Stout JL *et al.* (2000) An index for quantifying deviations from normal gait. *Gait and Posture* **11**:25–31.

Steven MM, Capell HA, Sturrock RD *et al.* (1983) The physiological cost of gait (PCG): a new technique for evaluating nonsteroidal antiinflammatory drugs in rheumatoid arthritis. *British Journal of Rheumatology* **22**:141–145.

Whittle MW. (1982) Calibration and performance of a three-dimensional television system for kinematic analysis. *Journal of Biomechanics* **15**:185–196.

Whittle MW. (1999) Generation and attenuation of transient impulsive forces beneath the foot: a review. *Gait and Posture* **10**: 264–275.

Whittle MW, Levine DF. (1997) Measurement of lumbar lordosis as a component of clinical gait analysis. *Gait and Posture* **5**:101–107.

Zijlstra W, Hof AL. (2003) Assessment of spatio-temporal gait parameters from trunk accelerations during human walking. *Gait and Posture* **18**: 1–10.

Zijlstra W, Rutgers AWF, Hof AL *et al.* (1995) Voluntary and involuntary adaptation of walking to temporal and spatial constraints. *Gait and Posture* **3**:13–18.

Applications of gait analysis

5

The aim of this chapter is to provide a broad overview of some of the ways in which gait analysis is used, particularly in a clinical setting. It is not intended to transform the reader into an expert on the subject. Anyone planning to use gait analysis in clinical decision making should read all the texts listed at the end of this chapter, attend one or more courses on the interpretation of gait analysis data, and if possible spend some time studying or working in a clinical gait laboratory.

The applications of gait analysis are conveniently divided into two main categories: *clinical gait assessment* and *gait research*. Clinical gait assessment has the aim of helping individual patients directly, whereas gait research aims to improve our understanding of gait, either as an end in itself or in order to improve medical diagnosis or treatment in the future. There is obviously some overlap, in that many people performing clinical gait assessment use it as the basis for research studies. Indeed, this is the way that most progress in the use of clinical gait assessment is made.

Davis (1988) pointed out that there are considerable differences between the technical requirements for clinical gait assessment and those for gait research. For example, an intrusive measurement system and a cluttered laboratory environment might not worry a fit adult, who is acting as an experimental subject, but could cause significant changes in the gait of a child with cerebral palsy. In gait research, it might be acceptable to spend a whole day preparing the subject, making the measurements and processing the data, whereas in the clinical setting patients often tire easily and the results are usually needed as quickly as possible. The requirements for accuracy are generally not as great in the clinical setting as they are in the research laboratory, so long as the measurement errors are not large enough to cause a misinterpretation of the clinical condition. However, it is essential that those interpreting the data appreciate the possible magnitude of any such errors.

Finally, the system must be able to cope with a wide variety of pathological gaits. It is much easier to make measurements on normal subjects than on those whose gait is very abnormal, which may explain why the literature of the subject is dominated by studies of normal individuals! A final and important point is that there is no value in using a complicated and expensive measurement system, unless it provides information which is useful and which cannot be obtained in an easier way.

Gait research may be divided into clinical and fundamental research, the former concentrating on disease processes and methods of treatment, the latter on methods of measurement and the advancement of knowledge in biomechanics, human performance and physiology. This text will concentrate on clinical gait assessment and leave further consideration of the subject of gait research for more specialized publications.

CLINICAL GAIT ASSESSMENT

Clinical gait assessment seeks to describe, on a particular occasion, the way in which a person walks. This may be all that is required, if the aim is simply to document their current status. Alternatively, it may be just one step in a continuing process, such as the planning of treatment or the monitoring of progress over a period of time.

Rose (1983) made a distinction between gait analysis and gait assessment. He regarded gait analysis as 'data gathering' and gait assessment as 'the integration of this information with that from other sources for the purposes of clinical decision making'. This usage of the term 'analysis' differs from that in more technical fields, in which it means 'the processing of data to derive new information'. However, Rose's use of the term is helpful, because it points out that gait assessment is simply one form of clinical assessment. Medical students are taught that clinical assessment is based on three things: history, physical examination and special investigations. In this context, gait analysis is simply a special investigation, the results of which will augment other investigations, such as x-ray reports and blood biochemistry, to provide a full clinical picture. The term 'gait evaluation' is sometimes used instead of gait analysis.

The simplest form of gait assessment is practiced every day in orthopedic, physical therapy and rehabilitation clinics throughout the world. Every time a doctor or therapist watches a patient walk up and down a room, they are performing an assessment of the patient's gait. However, such assessment is often unsystematic and the most that can be hoped for is to obtain a general impression of how well the patient walks, and perhaps some idea of one or two of the main problems. This could be termed an 'informal' gait assessment. To perform a 'formal' gait assessment requires a careful examination of the gait, using a systematic approach, if possible augmented by objective measurements. Such a gait assessment will usually produce a written report and the discipline involved in preparing such a report is likely to result in a much more carefully conducted assessment.

The gait analysis techniques which are used in clinical gait assessment vary enormously, with the nature of the clinical condition, the skills and facilities available in the individual clinic or laboratory and the purpose for which the assessment is being conducted. In general, however, clinical gait assessment is performed for one of three possible reasons: it may form the basis of clinical decision making, it may help with the diagnosis of an abnormal gait, or it may be used to document a patient's condition. Thesewill be considered in turn.

Clinical decision making

Both Rose (1983) and Gage (1983) suggested that clinical decision making in cases of gait abnormality should involve three clear stages.

1. *Gait assessment:* this starts with a full clinical history, both from the patient and from any others involved, such as doctors, therapists or family members. Where a patient has previously had surgery, details of this should be obtained, if possible from the operative notes. History taking is followed by a physical examination, with particular emphasis on the musculoskeletal system. In many laboratories, physical examinations are performed by both a doctor and a physical therapist. Finally, a formal gait analysis carried out.

2. *Hypothesis formation:* the next stage is the development of a hypothesis regarding the cause or causes of the observed abnormalities. Time needs to be set aside to review the data, and consultation between colleagues, particularly those from different disciplines, is extremely valuable. Indeed, almost all of those using gait assessment as a clinical decision-making tool stress the value of this 'team approach'. In forming a hypothesis as to the fundamental problem in a patient with a gait disorder, Rose emphasized that the patient's gait pattern is not entirely the direct result of the pathology, but is the net result of the original problem and the patient's ability to compensate for it. He observed that the worse the underlying problem, the easier it is to form a hypothesis, since the patient is less able to compensate.

3. *Hypothesis testing:* this stage is sometimes omitted, when there is little doubt as to the cause of the abnormalities observed. However, where some doubt does exist, the hypothesis can be tested in two different ways – either by using a different method of measurement or by attempting in some way to modify the gait. Some laboratories routinely use a fairly complete 'standard protocol', including video recording, kinematic measurement, force platform measurements and surface electromyography (EMG). They will

then add other measurements, such as fine wire EMG, where this is necessary to test a hypothesis. Other clinicians start the gait analysis using a simple method, such as video recording, and only add other techniques, such as EMG or the use of a force platform, where they would clearly be helpful. Rose (1983) opposed the use of a standard protocol for all patients, since some of the procedures turn out to have been unnecessary and there is a risk of ending up with 'an exhausted subject in pain'. The other method of testing a hypothesis is to reexamine the gait after attempting some form of modification, typically by the application of an orthosis to limit joint motion or by paralyzing a muscle using local anesthetic. The ultimate form of gait modification is the surgical operation, with retesting following recovery. However, this is a rather drastic form of 'hypothesis testing', which can be used only where there is a good reason to suppose that the operation will lead to a definite improvement.

Different types of gait analysis data may be useful for different aspects of the gait assessment. Information on foot timing may be useful to identify asymmetries and may indicate problems with balance and stability. The general gait parameters give a guide to the degree of disability and may be used to monitor progress or deterioration with the passage of time. The kinematics of limb motion describe abnormal movements, but do not identify the 'guilty' muscles.

The most useful measures are probably the joint moments and joint powers, particularly if this information is supplemented by EMG data. Hemiparetic patients may show greater differences between the two sides in muscle power output than in any of the other measurable parameters, including EMG. Winter (1985) stressed the need to work backwards from the observed gait abnormalities to the underlying causes in terms of the 'guilty' motor patterns, using both the EMG and the moments about the hip, knee and ankle joints. He offered a method of charting gait abnormalities and a table giving the common gait disorders, their possible causes and the type of evidence which would confirm or refute them (Table 5.1). Although the next step, that of treatment, was not considered in detail, he suggested that once an accurate diagnosis had been made, the therapist would be challenged to 'alter or optimize the abnormal motor patterns'.

Many others working in the field of clinical gait assessment have noted the difficulty of deducing the underlying cause from the observed gait abnormalities, because of the compensations which take place. A number of attempts have been made to simplify this process, by using a systematic approach. Computer-based expert systems are very suitable for this type of application and a number of such systems have been developed for clinical gait assessment. Since gait patterns are seldom clear cut, such expert systems cannot generally use a fixed set of rules but rather need to learn to recognize patterns within complex sets of data. Techniques such as neural networks and

Table 5.1 Common gait abnormalities, their possible causes and evidence required for confirmation (reproduced with permission from Winter, 1985)

Foot slap at heel contact	Below normal dorsiflexor activity at heel contact	Below normal tibialis anterior EMG or dorsiflexor moment at heel contact
Forefoot or flatfoot initial contact	(a) Hyperactive plantarflexor activity in late swing (b) Structural limitation in ankle range (c) Short step length	(a) Above normal plantarflexor EMG in late swing (b) Decreased dorsiflexor range of motion (c) See (a–d) immediately below
Short step	(a) Weak push off prior to swing (b) Weak hip flexors at toe off and early swing (c) Excessive deceleration of leg in late swing (d) Above normal contralateral hip extensor activity during contralateral stance	(a) Below normal plantarflexor moment or power generation (A2) or EMG during push off (b) Below normal hip flexor moment or power or EMG during late push off and early swing (c) Above normal hamstring EMG or knee flexor moment or power absorption (K4) late in swing (d) Hyperactivity in EMG of contralateral hip extensors
Stiff-legged weightbearing	Above normal extensor activity at the ankle, knee or hip early in stance*	Above normal EMG activity or moments in hip extensors, knee extensors or plantarflexors early in stance
Stance phase with flexed but rigid knee	Above normal extensor activity in early and mid-stance at the ankle and hip, but with reduced knee extensor activity	Above normal EMG activity or moments in hip extensors and plantarflexors in early and mid-stance
Weak push off accompanied by observable pull off	Weak plantarflexor activity at push off. Normal, or above normal, hip flexor activity during late push off and early swing	Below normal plantarflexor EMG, moment or power (A2) during push off. Normal or above normal hip flexor EMG or moment or power during late push off and early swing
Hip hiking in swing (with or without circumduction of lower limb)	(a) Weak hip, knee or ankle dorsiflexor activity during swing (b) Overactive extensor synergy during swing	(a) Below normal tibialis anterior EMG or hip or knee flexors during swing (b) Above normal hip or knee extensor EMG or moment during swing
Trendelenburg gait	(a) Weak hip abductors (b) Overactive hip adductors	(a) Below normal EMG in hip abductors: gluteus medius and minimus, tensor fascia lata (b) Above normal EMG in hip adductors, adductor longus, magnus and brevis, and gracilis

Note: there may be below normal extensor forces at one joint but only in the presence of abnormally high extensor forces at one or both of the other joints.

fuzzy logic are being explored for this purpose (Chau, 2001). No doubt the number and quality of such systems will increase in the future.

The following paragraphs describe how gait assessment is used for clinical decision making in a 'typical' laboratory. The details will, of course, differ from one laboratory to another, based on the skills and interests of the laboratory personnel, the facilities and equipment available, and the types of patient seen.

When the patient arrives at the facility, a thorough history is obtained and a physical examination is performed, by both a physician and a physical therapist. Height, weight and a number of other measurements are made. The patient's gait is video-recorded, viewing the patient from both sides and from the front and back. The 'technological' element of the gait analysis is performed, using a television/computer kinematic system and one or more force platforms. The number of cameras used is dictated largely by economics. Ideally, at least six cameras should be used but three can give acceptable data, particularly if measurements are made from only one side of the body at a time. Most laboratories record surface EMG, either on muscles which are selected on a case-by-case basis or on a standard set, such as gluteus maximus, quadriceps, medial and lateral hamstrings, triceps surae, tibialis anterior and the hip adductors. Depending on the clinical condition, fine wire EMG of selected muscles may be recorded, either at the same time or later. For example, Gage *et al.* (1984) reported that where a hip flexion contracture is present, their laboratory routinely records fine wire EMG from the iliopsoas. Some facilities record kinetic, kinematic and EMG data at the same time; others find it more convenient to record EMG separately.

Since great variability may exist between one walk and another, any single walk may not be representative, particularly if the patient hesitates or momentarily loses their balance. For this reason, a number of walks are recorded and the results examined for consistency. Depending on the clinical status of the patient, walks may be made under a number of different conditions, for example with and without shoes, with or without an orthosis, or using different walking aids.

Once preliminary reports on the history and physical examination have been prepared, the data processed and charts printed, the 'team' meets to discuss the case. The composition of the team varies considerably from one facility to another, but it would commonly consist of a physician, a physical therapist and a kinesiologist or bio-engineer, with the optional addition of other physicians, physical therapists, prosthetists and orthotists. Indeed, anyone with an interest in providing the best possible care for the patient may be invited to join the team to discuss a particular patient. In many facilities, the team includes the orthopedic surgeon who will ultimately perform any necessary surgery.

The assessment begins with a careful review of the patient's history and the physical examinations by the physician and physical therapist. The gait video recording is watched and discussed and notes are made for inclusion in a final report. The general gait parameters are noted, to determine the degree of disability and the effects of any changes in conditions, such as orthoses or walking aids. Different gait analysis systems provide different amounts of technical data on the patient's gait and examination of the 'charts' can be a long and painstaking process. One of the most important parts of the assessment is to identify deviations from normal in the joint angles and to determine the cause of such deviations. This process is easier if joint moments and powers are available. Joint moments indicate in general terms which structures in the region of a joint are coming under tension and the degree of tension in them. Joint powers may help to discriminate between concentric muscle contraction, eccentric muscle contraction and passive tension in soft tissues. They can also distinguish between powerful and weak muscle contractions. The EMG also contributes to this process, by identifying which muscles are electrically active and are thus candidates for developing tension, at different times during the gait cycle.

Very briefly, interpretation of the gait analysis charts may involve the following steps.

1. *Joint angle*: what is the angle of a joint at a particular part of the gait cycle and in which direction is it moving?
2. *Joint moment:* is the internal moment extensor or flexor? This will indicate what muscles or ligaments are under tension and to what degree.
3. *Joint power:* is power generation or absorption taking place? This would indicate concentric or eccentric contraction, or storage and release of energy by stretching elastic tissues.
4. *EMG:* is the muscle electrical activity consistent with the kinematic data?

At this time, a hypothesis is formed as to the detailed cause of any gait abnormalities present. This may indicate a need for further data, such as fine wire EMG recordings from other muscles (Fig. 5.1), and the patient may be asked to return for further tests. Having made a detailed diagnosis of the patient's functional problems, the team decides on an appropriate form of treatment, which in many cases involves surgery. In such cases, the final stage of assessment would be an 'examination under anesthetic', made just prior to the commencement of surgery. The muscle relaxant used with the anesthetic abolishes spasticity and makes it possible to distinguish between structural abnormalities, such as contractures, and the effects of muscle tension. If the treatment selected involves physical therapy or the use of an orthosis, the patient would be monitored during the course of such treatment, to determine whether the initial decisions were appropriate.

Once treatment has been carried out and after a suitable recovery period, a further gait assessment is often performed. The purpose of this is firstly to determine the success of the treatment and secondly to decide whether the

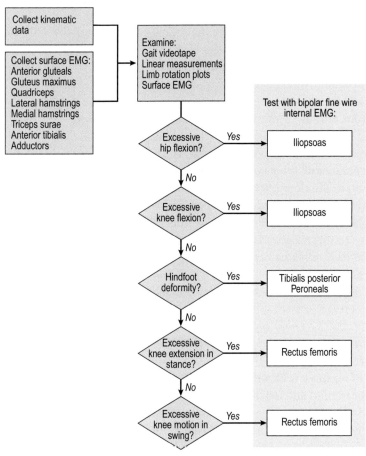

Fig. 5.1 Gait assessment flowchart, used for selecting muscles for testing with fine wire EMG (Davis, 1988).

patient would benefit from further surgery, physical therapy or the prescription of an orthosis. It also gives the clinical team the opportunity to perform a critical review of the original diagnosis and treatment plan, to decide whether the correct decisions were made. If an error has been made, it is important to recognize it and to learn from it, to prevent it from happening again. There is usually no change in EMG postoperatively and the main criteria for determining the success (or otherwise) of treatment are the general gait parameters and the joint rotations. In subjects in whom it can be measured from the kinematic data, the estimated external work of walking (EEWW) may also be used as a measure of improvement. According to Gage, total body energy consumption is the best measure of the success of treatment. Perry uses three criteria to gauge success: walking speed, energy consumption and cosmesis.

Diagnosis of abnormal gait

Most patients undergoing gait assessment have already been diagnosed, as far as the principal disease or condition affecting them is concerned. In such cases, gait assessment is carried out to make a more detailed diagnosis, relating to the exact state of particular joints and muscles. On occasion, however, a patient is seen in whom the cause of an abnormal gait is not clear.

A number of apparently abnormal gait patterns are, in fact, habits rather than the result of underlying pathology and the techniques of gait analysis may be useful to identify them. Since any pathology affecting the locomotor system generally reduces a person's ability to alter their gait pattern, a variable gait may be suggestive of a habit pattern and a highly reproducible gait may suggest a pathological process. However, the assessment must take many other factors into account, including the possibility of a pathological process which includes an element of variability, such as ataxia or athetosis.

One unusual application of gait analysis is to distinguish between a gait abnormality due to a genuine neuromuscular cause and one due to a psychogenic cause, such as may be seen in cases of malingering (Wesdock *et al.*, 2003).

An example of the use of gait assessment to differentiate between pathological gaits and habit patterns is in the diagnosis of toe walking. Some children prefer to walk on their toes, rather than on the whole foot, in a pattern known as 'idiopathic toe walking'. It is important, but also quite difficult, to be able to differentiate between this relatively harmless and self-limiting condition and more serious conditions, such as cerebral palsy. Hicks *et al.* (1988) stated that earlier attempts to establish the diagnosis, using EMG alone, had not been successful. In their study, they compared the gait kinematics of seven idiopathic toe walkers and seven children with mild spastic diplegia. There was a clear difference between the two groups in the pattern of sagittal plane knee and ankle motion. Both groups had initial contact either by the flat foot or by toe strike but in the case of the toe walkers, this was due to ankle plantarflexion, whereas in the children with cerebral palsy it was due to knee flexion. There were also other differences between the two groups, suggesting that gait assessment would be very helpful in making a differential diagnosis.

Documentation of a patient's condition

Although clinical decision making is the most direct way in which gait assessment may be used to help an individual patient, there are also instances when simply documenting the current state of a patient's gait may be of value. For some purposes, such documentation may be needed only on a single occasion, where the aim is to quantify a patient's disability. For other purposes, a series of gait assessments over a period of time may be used to monitor either progress or deterioration.

As part of the overall assessment of a patient with a disability, a clinician may require more detail about how well they walk. This type of gait assessment may be directly intended for use in clinical decision making, but it is sometimes performed speculatively, in case it should reveal a treatable cause for the patient's walking disorder.

Gait assessment is frequently used to document the progress of a patient undergoing some form of treatment. The results of the assessment may be used to identify areas where the treatment is ineffective or it may define an end point for stopping treatment, when progress appears to have ceased. Another use of this type of serial assessment is to convince the patient or their relatives that progress has been made, when their own faulty recollection tells them it has not. An objective form of monitoring progress is particularly important for use in the evaluation of novel and controversial methods of treatment, where the enthusiasm of the investigators has been known to lead to errors of judgment!

Gait assessment may form part of the overall documentation of a number of medical conditions that involve the locomotor system. A deterioration in gait with the passage of time may be detected early, allowing remedial action to be taken. It may also identify clinical signs which should be looked for in other cases of the same condition, particularly if it is very uncommon.

The shape of the ground reaction force curve is sometimes used empirically to monitor progress in rehabilitation. It has been observed that patients walking slowly and painfully have a flat-topped curve, which gradually changes towards the double-peaked normal curve (see Fig. 2.19) as their condition improves.

A regrettable but inescapable part of medical practice today is concerned with litigation. The ability of gait assessment to measure, objectively, at least some aspects of disability makes it very useful in supporting claims for damages. The author was the first person to present gait analysis data as evidence in a court of law in the United Kingdom, in a case in which a child suffered spastic hemiplegia as a result of a motor vehicle accident. Another aspect of litigation concerns medical practice itself and the risk that a doctor or other healthcare professional may be sued for negligence. Now that gait assessment has shown its value in the management of cerebral palsy, it may only be a matter of time before it is considered unwise to operate on a patient with cerebral palsy without a preoperative gait assessment.

CONDITIONS BENEFITING FROM GAIT ASSESSMENT

A large number of diseases affect the neuromuscular and musculoskeletal systems and may thus lead to disorders of gait. Among the most important are:

1. Cerebral palsy
2. Parkinsonism
3. Muscular dystrophy
4. Osteoarthritis
5. Rheumatoid arthritis
6. Lower limb amputation
7. Stroke
8. Head injury
9. Spinal cord injury
10. Myelodysplasia
11. Multiple sclerosis.

While it is possible that gait assessment may benefit a person affected by any one of these conditions, it is clear that greater benefits are possible in some pathologies than in others. This chapter will end with a consideration of those conditions for which there is good evidence that gait assessment is worthwhile.

Cerebral palsy

Since the management of individuals with cerebral palsy is, at present, the main clinical use for gait analysis, it has been given a chapter of its own (Chapter 6).

Gait disorders of the elderly

Cunha (1988) discussed the gait of the elderly and pointed out that many pathological gait disorders are incorrectly thought to be part of the normal aging process. Identification of an underlying cause, which may be treatable, could result in an improved life for the patient and a reduced risk of falls and fractures. Cunha classified the causes of the gait disorders of old age as follows: neurological, psychological, orthopedic, endocrinological, general, drugs, senile gait and associated conditions. He described the features of the gait in many conditions affecting the elderly and suggested a plan for the investigation and management of these patients.

Other conditions

A number of other possible uses for gait assessment in clinical decision making have been suggested over the years. In most cases, the publications dealing with these applications have been largely descriptive, with examples of clinical applications, such as the following.

Rose (1983) suggested that gait analysis was useful in the assessment of patients with multiple joint disease. He cited the case of a woman with a stiff but painless hip on one side and a painful deformed knee on the other. Gait analysis showed that the stiff hip was causing abnormal loading in the painful knee, suggesting that total knee joint replacement would be 'doomed to early failure'. The recommended course of action was to perform an operation to improve the mobility of the hip, before attempting any surgery on the knee. Rose did not, however, see any great value in performing gait assessment on patients requiring the replacement of only a single joint.

Prodromos *et al.* (1985) investigated the variable clinical results which follow the operation of high tibial osteotomy, for osteo-arthritis of the knee with a varus deformity. They found that clinical success or failure could be predicted by the preoperative measurement of the frontal plane moment of force at the knee, those patients with a high moment having a significantly worse result, with a recurrence of deformity, than those with a low moment.

Patients with a rupture of the anterior cruciate ligament in the knee may show altered muscle activity, for example an increase in the activity of the hamstrings. EMG of these muscles could be used either as a diagnostic aid or to monitor the results of ligament replacement surgery. Berchuck *et al.* (1990) reported a 'quadriceps avoidance' pattern, in which individuals with a ruptured anterior cruciate ligament lacked the normal internal knee extension moment provided by quadriceps contraction. Roberts *et al.* (1999) later challenged this finding, which may relate more to knee pain than to the absence of the anterior cruciate ligament.

The management of hemiplegia may be enhanced if a careful assessment of a patient's gait is performed. This may be used as a basis for planning either physical therapy (New York University, 1986) or some form of surgical treatment. Hemiplegic patients tend to walk very inefficiently, so that measuring their joint moments and powers may suggest ways in which training could be used to reduce their energy expenditure. Waters *et al.* (1979) used fine wire electrodes to measure the EMG activity of all four heads of the quadriceps muscle, in hemiplegic patients with a stiff-legged gait. If there was overactivity in only one or two components of the muscle, during late stance phase and early swing, good results were obtained by performing appropriate tenotomies.

Other neurological conditions could also benefit from the information provided by gait assessment. For example, Rose (1983) stated that gait assessment can make a significant contribution to the management of muscular dystrophy.

Lord *et al.* (1986) suggested that the measurement of pressure beneath the foot could play a useful part in patient management, by making it possible to provide custom-made pressure-relieving insoles. The manufacture of these insoles could be achieved either by a craftsman, using information provided by the measurement system, or automatically by some form of computer-aided design and manufacture (CAD-CAM). Having produced the insoles, further pressure measurement could then be used to check their effectiveness. Force platforms have also been used as an aid in the prescription of corrective footwear, by measuring the symmetry of the force patterns between the two feet. Pressure distribution beneath the foot could also be used to monitor the results of treatment for various types of foot disorder, such as a fracture involving the subtalar joint.

A high proportion of longstanding diabetics develop peripheral neuropathy and many of these go on to develop pressure sores on the feet. Regrettably, these may not be detected until deep-seated infection has occurred, which often leads to amputation and occasionally to death. The detection of these pressure sores does not need gait assessment – it merely needs someone to inspect the feet on a regular basis. However, the detection of high pressures, before ulceration has occurred, can be achieved by a pressure measurement system. Cavanagh *et al.* (1985) described a method which could be used to detect areas of dangerously high pressure beneath the feet of diabetic patients, prior to the actual formation of an ulcer.

Other groups of patients who might benefit from foot pressure monitoring are those with peripheral neuropathy from other causes, such as Hansen's disease (leprosy), and people with severely deformed feet, for example from rheumatoid arthritis.

In many other conditions affecting gait, the use of gait analysis gives a better insight into the exact nature of the deficit and the way in which the patient is able to compensate for it. This applies particularly where moments and powers have been measured. It may lead to a better understanding of the pathological condition itself and may also suggest improved methods of treatment. For example, if a patient is compensating for weakness of one muscle group by using other muscles, physical therapy could be aimed at strengthening those muscles and perhaps at increasing the patient's skill in using these slightly unnatural movements.

As well as its use in comparative trials between two or more forms of treatment, gait analysis is also commonly used simply to quantify the benefit which a patient receives from a particular type of treatment. In such cases, a comparison may be made with pretreatment data values for that patient and with comparable results from normal individuals. Figure 5.2 shows an example of how the operation of high tibial osteotomy was successful in eliminating an excessively high external adduction moment at the knee (Jefferson & Whittle, 1989).

Gait assessment may be of value in the disciplines of prosthetics and orthotics. The alignment and adjustment of prosthetic limbs may be improved using objective measurements of gait, particularly if repeat trials are performed with different adjustments. The prescription of orthoses may be improved if the gait is monitored with the patient wearing different types or configurations of orthosis, for example with different ankle alignments on an ankle–foot orthosis for drop foot (Lehmann et al., 1987). Trials of different orthoses may also form part of the process of hypothesis testing, described above (Õunpuu et al., 1996).

The design and prescription of orthoses tend to be much more an art than a science and a significant proportion of orthotic devices are regrettably not used by the patients for whom they are made. Gait analysis is able to provide an insight into the functioning of orthoses and to compare different designs. It may also permit improvements to be made to existing designs, such as the Saltiel anterior floor reaction orthosis (Harrington et al., 1984). Some objective studies of orthoses have failed to demonstrate that they have any significant mechanical effects. It then becomes arguable whether the devices

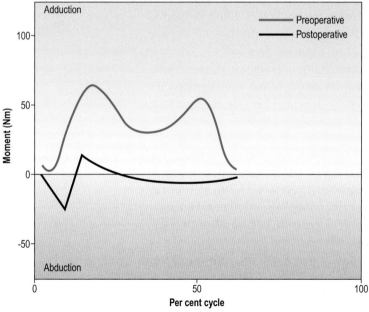

Fig. 5.2 Change in frontal plane external knee moment from excessive adduction moment to abnormally low biphasic moment, following high tibial osteotomy (Jefferson & Whittle, 1989).

really do have no effect, or whether their mode of action is too subtle for the methods of measurement being used.

Gait analysis can also be used for the assessment of new or modified forms of lower limb prosthesis. It may be used to examine the effects of changing the design of a prosthetic limb, such as by altering the mass distribution (Tashman *et al.*, 1985), or using knee joints with different types of braking mechanism (Hicks *et al.*, 1985). Two types of measurement are of particular value in this type of assessment: the kinematics of motion and the muscle moments and powers the amputee has to produce in order to be able to walk.

Measurement of the power output across the ankle joint is very valuable when comparing different prosthetic foot mechanisms. One of the major differences between the prosthetic foot and the natural foot is the inability of the prosthetic foot to generate power during pre-swing (third rocker). However, it is able to store energy during the second rocker and to release it during the third rocker, which may lead to a more natural gait pattern. Gait analysis can be used to examine the energy storage and recovery by prosthetic foot mechanisms and to determine how well particular types of foot suit different categories of patient. For example, a young subject who has suffered a traumatic amputation is much better able to take advantage of an energy-storing foot mechanism than an elderly subject who has received an amputation for vascular disease.

FUTURE DEVELOPMENTS

Gait analysis has advanced significantly since joint moments and powers have become routinely available. What would be of even more value, if it could be provided, would be knowledge of the forces in the different structures in and around the joints. The use of mathematical modeling permits estimates to be made of forces in tendons and ligaments and across articular surfaces. Unfortunately, a large number of unknown factors are involved, particularly the internal moments generated by different muscles and the extent of any co-contraction by antagonistic muscles. For this reason, such calculations can only be approximate but they may nonetheless be extremely valuable, particularly in clinical and biomechanical research. The output of mathematical models may be further refined using EMG. Most models offer a range of possible solutions, based on different combinations of active muscles. Even though it is not generally possible to convert EMG signals directly into muscle contraction force, the knowledge that a muscle is either inactive, contracting a little or contracting strongly may make it possible to eliminate at least some of the possible model solutions and thereby to improve the reliability of the results.

CONCLUSION

Gait analysis has had a long history and for much of this time it has remained an academic discipline with little practical application. This situation has now changed and the value of the methodology has been unequivocally demonstrated in certain conditions, particularly cerebral palsy. We are already seeing a decrease in the cost and complexity of kinematic systems and an increasing acceptance by clinicians of the results of gait analysis. This trend will hopefully continue, so that the use of these techniques will increase, both in those conditions for which its value is already recognized and in a variety of other conditions.

Although the current text has focused on gait analysis, this type of measurement equipment may also be used for other purposes – a fact which may be relevant to those trying to obtain funds to set up a gait analysis laboratory! The use of force platforms and kinematic systems for balance and posture testing has been referred to, as has their use in studying performance in a wide range of sports. Clinical studies have also been made of people standing up, sitting down, starting and stopping walking, ascending and descending stairs. The equipment has been used to measure the movements of the back, not only in walking but also in the standing and sitting positions. It has also been used to monitor the movements of the upper limbs, both in athetoid patients and in ergonomic studies of reach. Walking is only one of many things which can be done by the musculoskeletal system. It is only sensible to broaden our horizons and to use the power of the modern measurement systems to study a wide range of other activities.

References and suggestions for further reading

Berchuck M, Andriacchi TP, Bach BR *et al.* (1990) Gait adaptations by patients who have a deficient anterior cruciate ligament. *Journal of Bone and Joint Surgery* **72A**: 871–877.

Cavanagh PR, Hennig EM, Rodgers MM *et al.* (1985) The measurement of pressure distribution on the plantar surface of diabetic feet. In: Whittle M, Harris D (eds) *Biomechanical Measurement in Orthopaedic Practice*. Oxford: Clarendon Press, pp. 159–166.

Chau T. (2001) A review of analytical techniques for gait data. Part 1: fuzzy, statistical and fractal methods. *Gait and Posture* **13**: 49–66.

Cunha UV. (1988) Differential diagnosis of gait disorders in the elderly. *Geriatrics* **43**: 33–42.

Davis RB. (1988) Clinical gait analysis. *IEEE Engineering in Medicine and Biology Magazine* **September**: 35–40.

Gage JR. (1983) Gait analysis for decision-making in cerebral palsy. *Bulletin of the Hospital for Joint Diseases Orthopaedic Institute* **43**: 147–163.

Gage JR, Fabian D, Hicks R *et al.* (1984) Pre- and postoperative gait analysis in patients with spastic diplegia: a preliminary report. *Journal of Pediatric Orthopedics* **4**: 715–725.

Harrington ED, Lin RS, Gage JR. (1984) Use of the anterior floor reaction orthosis in patients with cerebral palsy. *Orthotics and Prosthetics* **37**: 34–42.

Hicks R, Tashman S, Cary JM *et al.* (1985) Swing phase control with knee friction in juvenile amputees. *Journal of Orthopaedic Research* **3**: 198–201.

Hicks R, Durinick N, Gage JR. (1988) Differentiation of idiopathic toe-walking and cerebral palsy. *Journal of Pediatric Orthopaedics* **8**: 160–163.

Jefferson RJ, Whittle MW. (1989) Biomechanical assessment of unicompartmental knee arthroplasty, total condylar arthroplasty and tibial osteotomy. *Clinical Biomechanics* **4**: 232–242.

Lehmann JF, Condon SM, Price R *et al.* (1987) Gait abnormalities in hemiplegia: their correction by ankle-foot orthoses. *Archives of Physical Medicine and Rehabilitation* **68**: 763–771.

Lord M, Reynolds DP, Hughes JR. (1986) Foot pressure measurement: a review of clinical findings. *Journal of Biomedical Engineering* **8**: 283–294.

New York University. (1986) *Lower Limb Orthotics.* New York: New York University Postgraduate Medical School.

Õunpuu S, Davis RB, DeLuca PA. (1996) Joint kinetics: methods, interpretation and treatment decision-making in children with cerebral palsy and myelomeningocele. *Gait and Posture* **4**: 62–78.

Prodromos CC, Andriacchi TP, Galante JO. (1985) A relationship between gait and clinical changes following high tibial osteotomy. *Journal of Bone and Joint Surgery* **67A**: 1188–1194.

Roberts CS, Rash GS, Honaker JT *et al.* (1999) A deficient anterior cruciate ligament does not lead to quadriceps avoidance gait. *Gait and Posture* **10**: 189–199.

Rose GK. (1983) Clinical gait assessment: a personal view. *Journal of Medical Engineering and Technology* **7**: 273–279.

Tashman S, Hicks R, Jendrzejczyk DJ. (1985) Evaluation of a prosthetic shank with variable inertial properties. *Clinical Prosthetics and Orthotics* **9**: 23–28.

Waters RL, Garland DE, Perry J *et al.* (1979) Stiff-legged gait in hemiplegia: surgical correction. *Journal of Bone and Joint Surgery* **61A**: 927–933.

Wesdock K, Blair S, Masiello G *et al.* (2003) Psychogenic gait: when it is and when it isn't – correlating the physical exam with dynamic gait data. Gait and Clinical Movement Analysis Society, Eighth Annual Meeting, Wilmington, Delaware, USA, pp. 279–280.

Winter DA. (1985) Concerning the scientific basis for the diagnosis of pathological gait and for rehabilitation protocols. *Physiotherapy Canada* **37**: 245–252.

Gait assessment in cerebral palsy

6

As early as 1983, Gordon Rose stated that decision making in cerebral palsy may be 'significantly affected' by the results of gait assessment (Rose, 1983). Concurring in this view, Gage (1983) suggested that the variable outcome following the surgical treatment of spastic diplegia was due to the fact that 'the spectrum of neurological pathology cannot be differentiated by clinical evaluation alone'. The assessment of individuals with cerebral palsy is now one of the most important applications of gait analysis (Õunpuu *et al.*, 1996).

Of the millions of people with cerebral palsy in the world, no more than a few thousand have received any systematic form of gait assessment prior to surgical treatment. However, the medical community is gradually coming to accept that better treatment decisions can be made with the benefit of gait assessment, and new gait labs are being opened all the time.

Much of this chapter is based on the book *The Treatment of Gait Problems in Cerebral Palsy* (Gage, 2004), publication details of which will be found in the bibliography. This should be required reading for anyone using gait analysis to plan treatment for locomotor problems in individuals with cerebral palsy. It details the practice of Gillette Children's Specialty Healthcare, St. Paul, Minnesota, USA – arguably the premier institution in the world for treating this condition.

BASIC PHYSIOLOGY OF MOVEMENT

All voluntary movement, including gait, commences with activity in several areas of the brain. This results in nervous impulses, which pass down the spinal cord and activate the motor nerves, which cause muscle contraction. Sensors in the muscles and surrounding structures provide feedback, which causes a modification of the pattern of movement. Three areas in the brain are particularly involved in this process.

1. The basal ganglia, which learn, and subsequently reproduce, basic movement patterns, known as *engrams*.
2. The motor cortex, which calls into action the necessary muscles and groups of muscles to perform the movements.
3. The cerebellum, which monitors the activity and provides feedback on whether or not it is being performed correctly.

The brainstem motor nuclei and spinal cord also take part in generating and controlling movements. Cerebral palsy may affect any or all of these areas and as a result may exist in many different patterns.

THE CAUSES OF CEREBRAL PALSY

The incidence of cerebral palsy in the USA is currently around 2 per 1000 live births. It is not a single disease but a collection of diverse clinical syndromes, which share a common origin – damage to the immature brain. Damage may occur in different areas of the brain, it may be extensive or localized and it may occur earlier or later in brain development. As a result, both the severity and the clinical pattern of cerebral palsy vary a great deal from one individual to the next. It is far more common in infants born prematurely than in those delivered at full term. The ultimate cause of the brain damage is a lack of oxygen in an area of the developing brain. This usually occurs through damage to the blood vessels, such as a hemorrhage or embolism, although it may also be caused by a drop in fetal blood pressure (du Plessis, 2004). The lack of oxygen damages or kills developing neurons, resulting in faulty functioning of part of the brain.

In many individuals, the cause of their cerebral palsy is not known; in other cases, the cause may be apparent, such as extreme prematurity or cerebral anoxia during a difficult delivery. Neonatal jaundice may also produce brain damage and subsequently cerebral palsy.

As well as the movement disorders associated with cerebral palsy, the brain damage often causes other problems, such as sensory or cognitive deficits, or epilepsy. The brain damage, once it has occurred, is static and will not get any worse. However, the clinical manifestations resulting from that brain damage will continue to develop and change as the child grows and matures. Treatment cannot (at present) do anything for the brain damage itself but it can prevent, or at least ameliorate, some of the worst secondary effects.

Cerebral palsy involves a loss of the selective control of muscles by the motor cortex and the emergence of spasticity and primitive patterns of contraction. As a general rule, the muscles are not weak but they may be unable to contract adequately at appropriate times in the gait cycle, due to a loss of coordination. Muscular contraction typically cannot be turned on or off rapidly and there is commonly a co-contraction of antagonists. Similar deficits are often seen in children or adults with traumatic brain injury.

Many people with cerebral palsy are incapable of walking. The majority of those who *are* able to walk have either spastic hemiplegia or spastic diplegia (both of which are described below). Since cerebral palsy is so variable, deciding what combination of treatments is best for an individual can be extremely difficult – hence the need for clinical gait assessment.

SPASTIC HEMIPLEGIA

Strictly speaking, *hemiplegia* implies a total paralysis on one side of the body and *hemiparesis* a partial paralysis, although the word 'hemiplegia' is often applied loosely to both conditions.

Spastic hemiplegia is the most common neurological cause of an abnormal gait. As well as occurring in cerebral palsy, it is also frequently seen in elderly people who have had a cerebrovascular accident ('stroke') and may also occur following traumatic brain injury. The characteristics of hemiparetic gait following a stroke were reviewed by Olney & Richards (1996). A companion paper (Richards & Olney, 1996) reviewed the natural history and treatment of the condition. Hemiplegic gait is characterized by spasticity and loss of function in some or all of the muscles of one side of the body, the other side being normal or nearly normal. The arms are usually affected more than the legs and people with hemiplegia generally walk with the affected arm held immobile, in a characteristic flexed posture. A person with hemiplegia usually possesses a mixture of normal motor control, spasticity and 'patterned responses', the exact combination depending on the severity and location of the brain damage (Perry, 1969). As well as the problems they experience with moving and controlling their limbs, many people with hemiplegia also have problems in maintaining balance, because a defect in the 'body image' causes them to ignore the affected side.

Since only one side of the body is affected, the majority of people with spastic hemiplegia are able to walk. Winters *et al.* (1987) showed that the gait pattern of children and young adults with this condition could be divided into four groups. These are numbered I to IV in order of increasing severity, each group having all the neurological deficits of the preceding one, with some additions. In general, the results of this study of young people agreed with other publications on the gait of elderly subjects following a cerebrovascular accident. Gage (1991) gave a very clear, illustrated account of this classification. Subsequent studies have confirmed the validity of the classification and provided information on the differences between the groups in terms of moments, powers and energy consumption. Stout *et al.* (1994) further refined this classification, dividing both group III and group IV into 'milder' and 'more severe' categories.

Group I subjects essentially have a single problem – a foot drop on the affected side. This causes initial contact to be by primary toestrike and also produces a functional increase in leg length during the swing phase. According to Winters et al. (1987), the plantarflexed attitude of the foot at initial contact leads to the use of several compensations: increased flexion of the knee and hip ('steppage') and an increased lumbar lordosis. The most common surgical treatment for this problem is to lengthen the Achilles tendon. However, this is unlikely to improve the gait, since the ankle is usually able to dorsiflex adequately. The significant problem in these individuals is the foot drop during the swing phase, caused by a relative weakness of the anterior tibial muscles, which can be treated adequately by a simple ankle–foot orthosis (AFO).

Group II subjects, as well as having a foot drop, have a static or dynamic contracture of the calf muscles, which holds the ankle in plantarflexion throughout the whole of the gait cycle. The difference in gait between group I and group II subjects is seen after mid-stance, when the persistent plantarflexion produces an external moment which forces the knee into hyperextension (the 'plantarflexion/knee extension couple'). According to Winters et al. (1987), advancement of the trunk is curtailed and the step length on the opposite side is decreased. As with the group I subjects, there is increased hip flexion with an associated increased lumbar lordosis. These people generally benefit from an operation to lengthen the Achilles tendon, as well as an orthosis to control the foot drop.

Group III subjects have a foot drop, contracted calf muscles and overactivity of both quadriceps and hamstrings. This causes a reduction in the total range of motion at the knee, with a marked reduction in swing phase flexion and a consequent increase in functional leg length. Since the opposite leg is usually fairly normal, many of these people respond by vaulting on the sound side (Gage, 1991). The other features of the group II pattern are also present: hyperextension of the knee in late stance, hip flexion and increased lumbar lordosis. Waters et al. (1979) showed that the stiff-legged gait is caused by an inappropriate contraction of one or more heads of the quadriceps (especially rectus femoris), during pre-swing and initial swing. Gage (1991) recommended hamstring lengthening, combined with transfer of the rectus femoris so that it acts as a knee flexor rather than an extensor.

The greatest degree of neurological involvement is seen in group IV subjects. In addition to the characteristics of the Group III subjects, they also have a reduced range of hip motion, due to overactivity of iliopsoas and the adductors. The hip is unable to extend fully, so anterior pelvic tilt and increased lumbar lordosis at the end of the stance phase are used to preserve the stride length. Full treatment of this condition includes lengthening the hip flexors (primarily psoas major), in addition to surgery to the muscles acting about the knee and ankle joints. The CD which accompanies this book includes data from an individual data from an individual with left sided spastic hemiplegia (Group IV).

SPASTIC DIPLEGIA

Spastic diplegia is another common manifestation of cerebral palsy. It primarily affects the legs, although there may be considerable asymmetry between the two sides. According to Gage (1991), most individuals with spastic diplegia are of normal intelligence. As its name suggests, spasticity is a particularly prominent element of this condition. The tension in the spastic muscles during development often leads to bony deformities, especially a torsion, or twisting, of the femur (femoral anteversion) and the tibia (external tibial torsion). A further significant problem in spastic diplegia is often a lack of stability in standing and walking. Many individuals with this condition continue to need walking aids, even after surgical treatment, to correct for deficiencies in balance. There is considerable variability between individuals, but the most common pattern consists of:

1. Hip flexion and internal rotation, due to overactivity by the iliopsoas, rectus femoris and hip adductors
2. Knee flexion, due to overactivity of the hamstrings, especially on the medial side
3. Equinus deformity of the foot and eversion of the hindfoot, due to overactivity by the triceps surae and peronei.

Excessive flexion of the hips leads to an increased lumbar lordosis, in order to get the femur as vertical as possible (see Fig. 3.8). The knee is held almost fixed by co-contraction of the hamstrings and quadriceps. Since the hamstrings are the more powerful of the two muscle groups, the knee remains flexed and its angle typically varies only between 30° and 40° of flexion. The equinus deformity of the foot causes a primary toestrike and loss of all three 'rockers' – plantarflexion in loading response, dorsiflexion in mid-stance and plantarflexion in pre-swing.

The hip, knee and ankle angles on the left side of a 6-year-old girl with spastic diplegia are shown in Fig. 6.1 (adapted from Gage, 1983). The hip angle, defined here as the angle between the femur and vertical, was fairly normal, although the pelvis was tilted forwards to compensate for tight hip flexors. The knee never extended beyond 25° of flexion, due to overactivity of the hamstrings. The plantarflexed position of the ankle throughout the cycle is evident, initial contact being made by the forefoot rather than the heel, because of spasticity of the triceps surae. Particularly striking on this plot is the very long stance phase and very short swing phase.

One difficulty in managing spastic diplegia is in determining the causes of inappropriate joint angles. For example, excessive hip flexion may be due to overactive hip flexors or to the anterior knee position caused by increased knee flexion – or both! Similarly, initial contact by the forefoot, rather than the heel, may be due to a static or dynamic ankle plantarflexion, or it may be the result

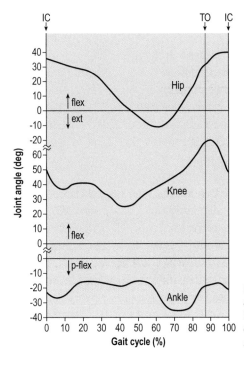

Fig. 6.1 Sagittal plane hip, knee and ankle angles during walking in the left leg of a 6-year-old girl with spastic diplegia (adapted from Gage, 1983). Abbreviations as in Fig. 2.5.

of the altered geometry caused by walking with a flexed knee. The functional leg length inequality caused by a lack of swing phase knee flexion commonly leads to a coping response, such as circumduction, hip hiking or vaulting. It is the aim of systematic gait analysis to determine the causes of the observed gait abnormalities and to use this information as the basis for planning treatment.

The pattern described above is not the only one seen in spastic diplegia, which is a highly variable condition. Significant numbers of people with spastic diplegia walk with hyperextension of the knee and a 'stiff-legged gait', which interferes with foot clearance during the swing phase.

OTHER VARIETIES OF CEREBRAL PALSY

As far as the clinical use of gait analysis is concerned, the most important categories of cerebral palsy are spastic hemiplegia and spastic diplegia, described above. *Spastic quadriplegia* affects all four limbs, the legs worse than the arms. Those who are affected by it are seldom able to walk, except in its milder forms, when the problems and approaches to treatment are similar to those described for spastic diplegia. Occasionally someone is seen who has all four limbs affected but the arms are worse than the legs. This condition is sometimes known as *double hemiplegia*. When both legs and one arm are principally involved, the term *triplegia* may be used.

The other major category in the classification of cerebral palsy involves the extrapyramidal system and includes abnormalities of movement such as *athetosis*, in which one or more limbs are 'waved about' in a seemingly random manner. People with such conditions seldom benefit from the use of gait analysis, which concentrates on the types of treatment used for spastic diplegia and hemiplegia (Gage, 1991).

CROUCH GAIT

An occasional complication of the treatment of cerebral palsy is the development of a *crouch gait* (Fig. 6.2), which may occur spontaneously (see below) but is particularly likely to occur if an equinus deformity of the foot is overcorrected, in the presence of a flexion contracture of the knee (Sutherland & Cooper, 1978). Excessive lengthening of the Achilles tendon may be caused directly by surgery or by postoperative stretching. The result is a calcaneus deformity of the foot, which keeps the line of the ground reaction force a long way behind the already flexed knee. This leads to a vicious circle in which the increased external moment leads to an increased force in the quadriceps, which gradually stretches the patellar tendon, further increasing the knee flexion and hence the external moment. Sutherland & Cooper (1978) stressed the need to correct the knee deformity before operating on the heel cord. Crouch gait may also occur in cerebral palsy without any operative intervention, as a result of spasticity of either the hip flexors or the hamstrings. The CD which accompanies this book includes data from an individual with crouch gait.

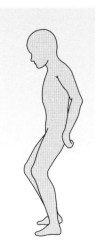

Fig. 6.2 Position of body at mid-stance in a 12-year-old child with crouch gait, following Achilles tendon lengthening for spastic diplegia (adapted from Sutherland & Cooper, 1978).

SPASTICITY

Spasticity is found in most (but not all) individuals with cerebral palsy and is often the dominant clinical feature (Peacock, 2004). It results from an increase in activity of the stretch reflex, described in Chapter 1 (p. 29), because of a decrease in the inhibitory nervous impulses passing down the upper motor neurons from the brain (Fig. 6.3). When a muscle is stretched, the stretch receptors within it send nerve impulses into the spinal cord, where they stimulate motor nerve fibers supplying the same muscle. Thus, stretching a muscle causes it to contract – the stretch reflex.

In normal individuals, the stretch reflex is not particularly active, because nervous impulses passing down the upper motor neurons from the brain inhibit it. When this inhibition is partly or wholly lost, the stretch reflex becomes hyperactive. A small reduction in inhibition leads to an exaggeration of the normal stretch reflex, such as a particularly vigorous 'knee jerk'. A major reduction, however, causes the muscle to become spastic, where it may show 'resting tone' (contraction when the individual is at rest) and where any attempt to stretch it, even slowly, causes it to respond with a strong contraction. The strength of the contraction increases with the speed at which the muscle is stretched, causing a 'velocity-dependent' reflex contraction.

Spasticity may result from brain damage in a number of areas but primarily involves the reticular and vestibular nuclei, which are in the

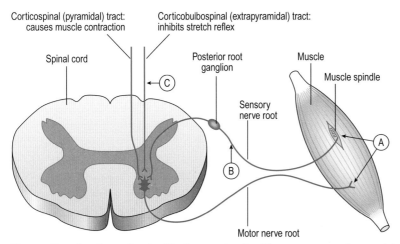

Fig. 6.3 Neural pathways involved in the stretch reflex. Three treatments for spasticity reduce the activity of the stretch reflex, acting at different locations. A: Botulinum toxin ('Botox') paralyzes numerous muscle fibers, including the intrafusal muscle fibers in the muscle spindle. B: Selective dorsal rhizotomy (SDR) reduces input to the stretch reflex, by removing some of the afferent nerve fibers from the muscle spindle. C: Baclofen increases the effectiveness of the inhibition of the stretch reflex which is provided by the extrapyramidal tract.

brainstem and form part of the 'extrapyramidal' system. The functional consequences of spasticity are:

1. A brake on movement
2. Impaired voluntary control
3. Reduced muscle stretch and hence growth
4. Abnormal bone growth due to resting tone.

LEVER ARM DYSFUNCTION

An understanding of joint moments is essential for those practicing gait analysis, because of their central role in locomotion. The main function of muscles is to generate moments, either to oppose other moments (generated by gravity, inertia or other muscles) or to initiate and maintain limb movement. In order for a muscle to generate a moment, three things are needed:

1. Muscle contraction
2. A rigid lever arm
3. A functional fulcrum (or pivot point).

Many of the abnormalities of gait in cerebral palsy are due to an inadequate lever arm, often due to bony deformity. Such problems have been dubbed 'lever arm dysfunction', which is defined as 'a set of conditions in which internal and/or external lever arms become distorted because of bony or positional deformities' (Gage & Schwartz, 2004). Five types of lever arm dysfunction have been described:

1. Short
2. Flexible
3. Malrotated
4. Abnormal pivot
5. Positional.

Short lever arms include actual shortening, such as mid-foot amputation, and functional shortening, where deformity leads to a reduced perpendicular distance for the lever arm, even though the length of a bony segment is normal, such as occurs in coxa valga.

The most common flexible lever arm is seen in flexible pes valgus, where the foot bends when force is applied, instead of remaining rigid and generating a moment. The reduced (internal) plantarflexion moment can lead to excessive knee flexion, through a failure to produce an adequate plantarflexion/knee extension couple.

Malrotation of a lever includes the 'malignant malrotation syndrome', where there is femoral anteversion, internal femoral torsion and external tibial torsion. The femoral rotation reduces the length of the quadriceps lever arm in the sagittal plane and hence reduces the magnitude of the (internal) knee extension moment; it also produces unwanted moments in the frontal and transverse planes. The external tibial torsion results in a center of pressure through the forefoot which is more posterior and more lateral than normal, again with a reduction in the 'primary' moment and the presence of unwanted 'secondary' moments.

An abnormal pivot is seen in hip subluxation or dislocation; muscle contraction displaces the femur relative to the pelvis, instead of generating a moment.

Positional abnormalities include conditions such as crouch gait, in which the anatomy may be fairly normal but the joints are abnormally flexed or extended, leading to an inappropriate length for a muscle lever arm.

An examination of the moments of force about the joints explains some of the gait abnormalities in cerebral palsy, since deformity may reduce the muscle lever arms, requiring very high muscle forces to be produced in order to produce modest joint moments.

GAIT PATTERNS IN CEREBRAL PALSY

The characteristics of cerebral palsy were given by Gage (1991) as follows:

1. Loss of selective muscle control
2. Dependence on primitive reflex patterns for ambulation
3. Abnormal muscle tone
4. Relative imbalance between muscle agonists and antagonists across joints
5. Deficient equilibrium reactions.

There is considerable variation between one individual and another in the way in which cerebral palsy affects the positions and movements of the joints. The clinical picture depends on which muscles are affected and on the timing of their contraction during the gait cycle (Gage & Schwartz, 2004).

The features of pathological gait can be divided into three forms of abnormality: primary, secondary and tertiary. The primary abnormality in cerebral palsy is brain injury and its direct results, including abnormal tone, loss of selective motor control and problems with balance. Such effects are normally permanent and little can be done to treat them. Secondary abnormalities include abnormal bone growth, muscle growth and joint alignments, including hip dislocation or subluxation and foot deformities, which result from limb development in the presence of abnormal forces. Some of these abnormalities are amenable to treatment. Tertiary abnormalities are the compensations that the subject makes to overcome the problems caused by the primary and secondary abnormalities. They often comprise the most 'visible' gait abnormalities, such as vaulting or circumduction. Such compensations are often vital to the subject and need to be carefully protected. If successful treatment of secondary abnormalities means that these compensations are no longer required, they will generally disappear.

Primary abnormalities affect three different aspects of gait: selective motor control, tone and balance. Selective motor control affects distal muscles more than proximal and biarticular muscles more than monarticular; better surgical results have been obtained from lengthening biarticular muscles (such as psoas and gastrocnemius) than their monarticular counterparts (iliacus and soleus). The most common abnormal tone is spasticity, which is velocity dependent. It acts as a brake on movement, interferes with voluntary control of movement and produces skeletal deformity. The use of a baclofen pump (see below) to reduce spasticity is an exception to the general rule that primary abnormalities cannot be treated. The primary abnormality of poor balance is almost always present in individuals with cerebral palsy; a good test for it is whether a person can stand on one leg for 10 seconds. Walking aids are extremely helpful for those with balance problems, but they may be inconvenient and unsightly and they increase energy expenditure.

Foot, knee and hip problems

The main problem seen at the foot in cerebral palsy is a loss of stability in stance. This may be caused in a number of different ways but most commonly by the foot being in equinus, due to the triceps surae overpowering the dorsiflexors. Contact between the foot and the ground is further forward than normal, resulting in an exaggerated plantarflexion/knee extension couple. Deformity of the foot usually develops, this being dynamic at first but later becoming fixed. The actual deformity varies with the type of cerebral palsy. Typically, in hemiplegia, the foot is in equinovarus. In diplegia and hemiplegia, the most common condition is the 'mid-foot break', in which there is extreme mobility between an equinus hindfoot and a supinated and abducted forefoot. In the swing phase of gait, foot deformity may cause difficulties with ground clearance or it may lead to poor positioning of the foot at initial contact (Gage, 2004, pp. 205-216). The CD which accompanies this book includes data from an individual with bilateral equinus.

Knee function is almost always compromised in cerebral palsy. The knee is frequently not aligned to the plane of progression and lever arm dysfunction is often present. The knee is often flexed at initial contact, which may cause ground contact by the forefoot instead of the heel. This may cause premature contraction of the gastrocnemius, which leads to a 'bounce gait', with excessive energy consumption. If the knee remains abnormally flexed throughout the stance phase (Fig. 6.4), the normal plantarflexion/knee

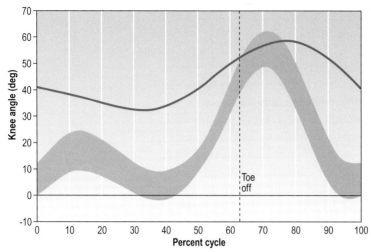

Fig. 6.4 Typical sagittal plane knee angle in spastic diplegia. Flexion is positive, and the normal adult range is given in pale blue. The knee is flexed at initial contact, extends a little during stance, and flexes a little during swing.

extension couple is lost and the internal knee extension moment has to be provided by quadriceps contraction, again with an increased energy consumption. In cerebral palsy, knee flexion in swing is very often delayed and reduced in magnitude. There are a number of reasons for this, including rectus femoris spasticity, reduced cadence and inadequate plantarflexion in pre-swing.

When the hip is involved in cerebral palsy, there is commonly a failure to remodel the anteversion present at birth, which causes a malrotation type of lever arm dysfunction. Two other causes of lever arm dysfunction in the hip, mentioned above, are coxa valga and subluxation or dislocation of the hip joint. Weakness of the hip extensors and abductors is common and may lead to the use of coping responses such as backward or lateral shifting of the trunk during the stance phase. Since little power can normally be generated at the ankle in cerebral palsy, increased power has to be generated at the hips and sometimes also at the knee.

Kinematic and kinetic patterns in cerebral palsy

The use of kinetic/kinematic systems for gait analysis, combined with ambulatory EMG, has led to the identification of a number of distinctive patterns in the joint angles and kinetics of individuals with cerebral palsy (Õunpuu, 2004). The detailed description of these patterns is beyond the scope of this introductory text, but some of the most obvious ones will be described briefly.

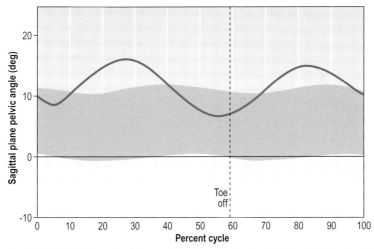

Fig. 6.5 'Double bump' pelvic angle in the sagittal plane (pelvic tilt). Anterior tilt is positive, and the normal adult range is given in pale blue. Anterior tilt is maximal in the middle of stance and swing, and minimal during double support.

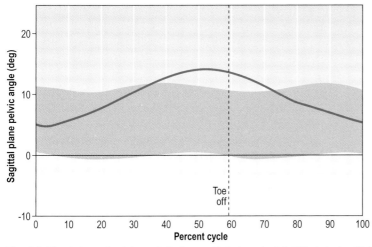

Fig. 6.6 'Single bump' pelvic angle in the sagittal plane (pelvic tilt). Anterior tilt is positive, and the normal adult range is given in pale blue. Anterior tilt increases during stance and decreases during swing, following flexion and extension of the hip joint.

The 'double bump pelvic pattern' (Fig. 6.5) occurs when the pelvis moves into anterior tilt at mid-stance on each side and into posterior tilt during double support. It occurs when the hip flexors are spastic and the hamstrings weak, on both sides. When one side is more affected than the other, a 'single bump pelvic pattern' (Fig. 6.6) may be seen, the pelvis following the movement of the femur on the more affected side; as the pelvis moves with one femur, the hip range of motion on that side is decreased, while that on the opposite side is increased.

Internal rotation of the hip, due to persistent anteversion, is a commonly seen pattern and may be combined with an internally rotated foot position. Internal rotation of the foot may be also be due to tibial torsion.

As well as a 'double bump' pattern of the pelvis, a 'double bump ankle pattern' (Fig. 6.7) may be seen, in which dorsiflexion in early stance is followed by plantarflexion, then further dorsiflexion. It is due to the reflex contraction of spastic plantarflexors, after they have been stretched at initial contact, and may include an element of clonus. This abnormality may be visible as a 'bounce gait'.

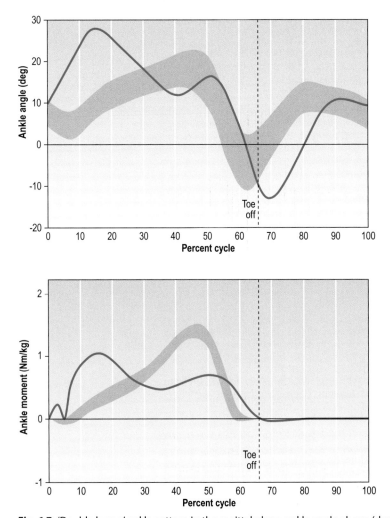

Fig. 6.7 'Double bump' ankle pattern in the sagittal plane; ankle angle above (dorsiflexion positive) and moment below (internal plantarflexion moment positive). Normal adult ranges are given in pale blue. During the first half of the stance phase, dorsiflexion stimulates spastic plantarflexors to contract, and thereby reduce the dorsiflexion. The pattern is repeated during the second half of stance.

Crouch gait (described above and illustrated on the CD accompanying this book) is a common problem in cerebral palsy. It is characterized by knee flexion throughout the gait cycle and has a number of different causes, including soleus weakness following selective dorsal rhizotomy or Achilles tendon lengthening. The opposite problem, excessive hyperextension of the knee, is also sometimes seen; it generally relates to equinus deformity and an excessive plantarflexion/knee extension couple.

As well as existing in isolation, patterns for single joints may be combined in various ways and may involve abnormalities in other planes. For example, a reduced range of hip flexion/extension (sagittal plane) may be compensated by an increased range of pelvic motion in the transverse plane – an exaggeration of the first determinant of gait. The reader is referred to more specialized publications, such as Gage (2004), for further details of these complex patterns.

GAIT ASSESSMENT

Gait assessment in the management of cerebral palsy takes place in three stages: gathering information, developing a problem list and developing a solution list. The gathering of information usually starts with history taking, physical examination and visual examination of the gait. These procedures are then followed by a more 'technical' examination, including kinematic and kinetic analysis, ambulatory electromyography and sometimes the measurement of energy expenditure. These methods are described in the following sections.

History taking

Both history taking and physical examination make important contributions to clinical gait evaluation, the overall aim of which is to identify three things: structural problems, functional problems and gait compensations. 'In order to prepare treatment plans and accurately assess outcomes of treatment, a balanced combination of history, detailed physical examination, observational gait analysis and computerized gait analysis must be interpreted together' (Trost, 2004). A detailed history includes the condition at birth and the age at which different milestones were passed. It also includes the current functional ability of the subject, such as how far they can walk and whether they can perform other activities, such as climbing stairs. Of particular importance is information on any treatments the individual has received. Where surgery has been performed, it is important to obtain operative reports, since the individual and their family may have an inadequate understanding or recollection of what was found and what was done.

Physical examination

The physical examination that forms part of clinical gait evaluation is extremely detailed and is well beyond the scope of the present volume. In order not to omit parts of the examination, it is essential to follow a standard protocol and most centers performing such assessments have developed a form or checklist for this purpose. The tests listed on the form used by Gillette Children's Specialty Healthcare have six main goals (Trost, 2004):

1. To determine strength and selective motor control of isolated muscle groups
2. To evaluate muscle tone and the influence of positional changes on tone
3. To estimate the degree of static deformity and/or muscle contracture at each joint
4. To assess torsional and other deformities of the bone
5. To describe fixed and mobile foot deformities
6. To assess balance, equilibrium responses and standing posture.

Muscle assessment is particularly aimed at determining strength and degree of control, especially the ability to isolate certain movements. When abnormal tone is present, it is important to distinguish between spasticity and dyskinesia (abnormal movement patterns), since the results of treatment are much more consistent for spasticity than for dyskinesia. Where limitations to joint range of motion are present, an attempt is made to distinguish between static (fixed) deformity, due to structural changes, and dynamic deformity due to muscle tone. In some cases, this distinction can only be made by examination under anesthetic, usually performed immediately before surgery. Special tests have been developed for differentiating monarticular and biarticular muscle tightness.

A number of special tests are also used to identify bony deformities, especially torsion of the long bones. A common deformity in spastic diplegia is femoral anteversion, which causes the individual to internally rotate the femur and hence the lower limb, and also to anteriorly tilt the pelvis. Other common problems include patella alta, tibial torsion and abnormal foot geometry. Foot examination includes identifying alignments between the leg and the hindfoot and between the hindfoot and the forefoot. Clinical examination of the foot may be supplemented by x-rays and by making close-up videos of the individual walking, supplemented where appropriate by braces or wedges. In the normal foot, hindfoot valgus and forefoot pronation occur during loading response, to provide shock absorption, and hindfoot varus and forefoot supination occur during pre-swing, to provide a rigid lever for propulsion. Deformities of the foot are likely to interfere with these normal functions. Computerized gait analysis typically provides little information on the functioning of the foot and this information must be supplied by clinical examination and testing.

Observational gait analysis

Despite the recent advances in computerized gait analysis, the visual examination of a subject's gait continues to be at least as important in their clinical assessment. For several decades past, visual examination has been supplemented by the use of cine photography, videotape or computerized video recording. By slowing down the subject's movements during gait, such methods make it much easier to visualize the different parts of the gait cycle and to identify subtle deviations from normal. Despite many years working in the field of gait analysis, the author cannot reliably identify stance phase knee flexion when watching a person walking at normal speed, although it is easy to see it when viewed in slow motion. As well as slowing the motion, videotape (or its equivalent) provides the opportunity to view the same walk many times, so that the major joints can be examined separately.

Whether using direct observation or video recording, visual gait analysis must be performed systematically, each joint being examined in turn for the presence or absence of both normal and pathological movements. A number of protocols and recording methods for this process have been published, including the widely used Rancho Los Amigos observational gait analysis form (Perry, 1992). The subject should be viewed (or 'filmed') from both sides, to identify sagittal plane abnormalities, and from the front and back, to identify frontal plane abnormalities; transverse plane abnormalities are most easily identified using computerized kinematic analysis.

Electromyography

The methodology of dynamic electromyography (EMG) has been described in Chapter 4 (p. 154). It is one of the most important tools in the assessment of the individual with cerebral palsy, both to pinpoint 'guilty' muscles and to decide whether a muscle is suitable for transplantation. Typically, surface electrodes are used for large muscles, or groups of muscles that tend to contract together, whereas fine wire electrodes are used for small muscles, such as tibialis posterior, or for muscles which are too deep for reliable surface recording, such as iliopsoas.

As early as 1977, Baumann & Hanggi showed that gait assessment using EMG could distinguish between muscle paralysis and incorrect phasing of muscle contraction. This becomes important when considering transplanting a muscle tendon to another site, to replace a muscle action which is deficient. This can be a very useful method of treatment in cerebral palsy, but it is vital to know the phasic activity of a muscle before transplanting it. As a general rule, the phasic activity of muscles in cerebral palsy is fixed, with no possibility of 're-education', so that if muscle activity is required during the stance phase, the surgery will be doomed to failure if the transposed muscle is only active during swing.

Gage *et al.* (1987) reported good results from an operation to correct the stiff-legged gait seen in some children with cerebral palsy. The operation, which was first suggested by Perry (1987), involves transfer of the rectus femoris to behind the knee, on either the medial or the lateral side (Chung *et al.*, 1997), in connection with lengthening of the hamstrings. Dynamic EMG is essential to identify those who would benefit from the procedure, which is appropriate only for those in whom there is contraction of the quadriceps throughout the swing phase.

In cerebral palsy, muscles often receive inappropriate neural stimulation from the damaged centers in the brain, resulting in longer periods of contraction and shorter (or absent) periods or relaxation. Because the fiber type of a muscle is determined by the pattern of stimulation it receives (Chapter 1, p. 28), this prolonged stimulation causes the muscles to predominate in type I (slow-twitch) fibers and for the muscles to be weaker than in normal individuals of the same age, where there would be a higher proportion of type II (fast-twitch) fibers.

The interpretation of EMG recordings from individuals with cerebral palsy is highly skilled and may be the most important single factor in choosing between treatment options. Since EMG is notoriously unreliable at estimating the *strength* of muscular contraction, interpretation is centered on examining the *timing* of contraction. In contrast, it may be possible to infer the strength of contraction from the kinetic data, showing how gait assessment draws together information from different sources, to provide a full picture of neuromuscular activity. EMG is particularly important in identifying the cause of a stiff-knee gait; individuals whose rectus femoris activity is predominantly during the swing phase of gait respond better to the rectus femoris transfer procedure than those with other patterns of activity (Miller *et al.*, 1997). Dynamic EMG is also of great value in distinguishing between various possible causes of varus foot deformity and recurvatum of the knee.

Energy expenditure

An important consequence of the increased tone and gait abnormalities of cerebral palsy is an increase in energy consumption. The physiological cost index (PCI), described in Chapter 4 (p. 159), is a fairly reliable indicator of metabolic activity in normal individuals, but it has been found unreliable in cerebral palsy. Where energy expenditure is a concern, it is better to measure oxygen uptake, which is routinely done in gait assessment at Gillette Children's Specialty Healthcare (Stout & Koop, 2004), although few other centers make such measurements. In children with cerebral palsy, oxygen cost (which relates energy consumption to the distance traveled) may be up to three times that of normal children of the same age.

The causes of increased energy consumption are many, including metabolic activity in spastic muscles and abnormal movements resulting from either joint contractures or 'lever arm disease'. The 'Normalcy Index' (Schutte *et al.*, 2000), which is increasingly used in the assessment of individuals with cerebral palsy, has been found to correlate with the oxygen cost of walking. The increased oxygen consumption in cerebral palsy is usually combined with a decreased maximum aerobic capacity (VO_2 max), which is the highest rate at which oxygen can be consumed during voluntary activity. Any activity in such individuals thus represents a greater proportion of their total capacity and makes them much more liable to fatigue. The energy cost of walking has been found to increase from the mildest (group I) hemiplegia to the most severe (group IV). It also increases from spastic diplegia to triplegia and further to quadriplegia. Children who use an assistive device use more energy than those who do not, for two reasons: the additional weight and movements involved in the use of an assistive device increase energy consumption, and children who need to use an assistive device are generally more affected than those who do not.

Future developments in gait assessment

Decisions on treatment are currently based on a detailed gait evaluation and the experience of the team, knowing which strategies are most likely to succeed in a given individual. However, in the future it may be possible to define a mathematical model of the musculoskeletal system, tailored to an individual person, and to use it to predict the results of different treatments (Arnold & Delp, 2004). Such models are already able to provide insights into the workings of the musculoskeletal system in cerebral palsy. For example, models have predicted that internal rotation in crouch gait may be due to the altered line of action of gluteus medius, rather than to the hamstrings or hip adductors. Modeling may also be used to predict joint moments and ranges of motion following lengthening of soleus and/or gastrocnemius for equinus contracture. It may also help to distinguish between different causes of a gait abnormality. For example, stiff-knee gait is often caused by overactivity of rectus femoris during the swing phase and responds well to the surgical procedure of rectus transfer, mentioned above. However, modeling may reveal other causes, such as a low angular velocity at toe off, which would not respond to the same procedure.

OVERVIEW OF TREATMENT

The treatment of cerebral palsy is a hugely complicated subject, clearly beyond the scope of an introductory book on gait analysis. What follows is a very brief review of the main forms of treatment. Readers involved in treating individuals with cerebral palsy should refer to more detailed and authoritative sources, such as Gage (2004), which provided most of the information given below.

It is essential in cerebral palsy, and indeed in other pathologies, to distinguish between the primary pathology and the 'coping responses'. A significant proportion of children undergoing surgery for cerebral palsy are made worse rather than better, because inappropriate treatment removes their ability to compensate. For example, a child may be vaulting on one side because of an inability to flex the opposite knee in the swing phase. If the vaulting is erroneously ascribed to a tight heel cord and treated by a heel cord lengthening, the gait is made worse, not better. Regrettably, errors of this type are all too common, particularly when treatment is prescribed without the benefit of gait assessment. Õunpuu *et al.* (1996) stated that joint kinetics (moments and powers) are helpful in distinguishing between the primary problem and secondary adaptations.

Realistic goal setting for the individual with cerebral palsy needs to concentrate on the final result, as an adult. In the past, surgical procedures have been performed which have improved walking in a child, but which turned out to be detrimental in the long run. For this reason, when any procedure is contemplated, the effects of growth must be taken into account. Realistic goals for individuals with athetoid cerebral palsy include communication and activities of daily living, but do not usually include walking. Some children with spastic quadriplegia are able to walk, but the majority cannot. In contrast, diplegia and hemiplegia are usually consistent with walking. However, in the past, such children have often lost a lot of their childhood by undergoing multiple surgical procedures, sometimes as much as once a year ('the birthday syndrome'), with ongoing physical therapy between operations. The current approach is to combine as many procedures as possible into a single operative session, known as 'multiple lower extremity procedures' (MLEP), thereby greatly reducing the number of hospital admissions. Although there are considerable benefits to an individual from having all their operations at once, there is also a risk that it will 'increase the likelihood of a judgment error' (Gage *et al.,* 1987). For this reason, MLEP can only be used safely if accurate and complete diagnostic information is available, based on a very thorough gait assessment.

Development is carefully monitored from the age of 1 year. Deformity is limited using orthoses, stretching casts and tone-reducing drugs (either oral or injected). Between the ages of 5 and 8, a careful review is performed to decide whether something needs to be done to reduce spasticity (see below). Spasticity reduction by itself is seldom sufficient, and once it has been performed and the child's gait has stabilized, a detailed gait assessment is performed to determine what further treatment is needed. The key to successful treatment is to use a combination of methods, tailored to the needs of the individual.

As has been stated previously, the individual with cerebral palsy faces a number of limitations, including impaired control of movement, spasticity, muscle and joint contractures, and bony deformity. Muscle contractures occur because spasticity and impaired motor control limit movement patterns, so that muscles do not get stretched to their full extent. Bony deformity occurs because the bones develop in an environment of increased and abnormal forces, due to spasticity and muscle contractures. Little can generally be done to improve motor control, but four principal options are available for the reduction of spasticity:

1. Oral medication (several possible drugs, including diazepam and baclofen)
2. Direct injection into muscles (botulinum toxin, phenol)
3. Dorsal rhizotomy
4. Implanted baclofen pump.

In the growing child, spasticity reduction should be combined with some form of muscle stretching, such as serial casting, splinting or range of motion exercises.

Oral medication is inexpensive and easy to administer, but it affects muscles throughout the body and often produces sedation. Direct injection of botulinum toxin ('Botox') is especially effective because it paralyzes the intrafusal muscle fibers (see Chapter 1, p. 29) as well as the main body of the muscle (Fig. 6.3A). However, it is expensive, toxicity limits its use to only a few muscles at any one time (typically four) and the effects wear off in 3–4 months. Phenol injections are inexpensive, but they may damage sensory nerves as well as motor; the effects may last as long as a year. It may be appropriate to treat some muscles with botulinum toxin and others (especially those with less sensory fibers) with phenol.

The surgical procedure of selective dorsal rhizotomy (SDR) is both difficult to perform and expensive, but it often gives a very useful reduction in spasticity. It acts by reducing the sensory input to the reflex arc (Fig. 6.3B). The procedure is contraindicated in those who rely heavily on spasticity to provide support, especially for transfers, since it will make them significantly weaker. Following SDR, it is usual to provide extensive physical therapy, including muscle stretching, strengthening and teaching coordinated activities.

The administration of baclofen intrathecally (into the space around the spinal cord), by an implanted pump, is also an important part of current treatment. Baclofen increases the level of descending inhibition acting on the reflex arc (Fig. 6.3C). Unlike SDR, its effects are reversible and it is free of the systemic effects of oral baclofen. However, it is expensive and, as with any implanted device, there is a possibility of complications.

The surgical treatment of individuals with cerebral palsy has five main aims (Novacheck, 2004):

1. The reduction of spasticity
2. The restoration of normal bony lever arms
3. The preservation of power generators
4. The correction of contractures
5. The simplification of the control system.

SUMMARY

The neurological deficit in cerebral palsy is permanent and irreparable, so that the timing of muscular contraction cannot be altered by treatment. However, the gait of a person with cerebral palsy can often be improved in other ways. The treatment of gait deviations in cerebral palsy can be divided into two main strategies: to decrease abnormal muscle forces (mainly by tendon lengthening, tendon transfer and botulinum toxin) and to increase useful forces (mainly by exercise, orthoses and osteotomies). The main forms of treatment are:

1. Using dorsal rhizotomy to reduce muscle tone, by destroying a proportion of the sensory fibers before they enter the spinal cord
2. Changing the mode of action of a muscle by tendon transplantation, e.g. changing rectus femoris into a knee flexor
3. Correcting bony misalignments, e.g. tibial or femoral rotational osteotomy
4. Strengthening a muscle by training
5. Making a muscle weaker or non-functional by lengthening or cutting its tendon, e.g. Achilles tendon lengthening
6. Lengthening a muscle by stretching, using serial casting and/or night splints
7. Lengthening a muscle by stretching, after paralyzing it by an injection of botulinum toxin or phenol (the effects of which last for several months), often combined with serial casting
8. Using an orthosis to limit the movement of a joint or to apply a force in a particular direction, e.g. ankle–foot orthosis (AFO) to control foot drop
9. Using drug treatment to reduce spasticity, e.g. oral baclofen

10. Using an implanted pump to infuse drugs into the space around the spinal cord, to reduce spasticity, e.g. intrathecal baclofen.

The management of individuals with cerebral palsy, with the aid of gait analysis, has developed considerably since about 1980 and it has an extensive literature of its own, which should be consulted for further information. The references below should provide a suitable entry point into this literature.

References and suggestions for further reading

Arnold AS, Delp SL. (2004) The role of musculoskeletal models in patient assessment and treatment. In: Gage JR (ed.) *The Treatment of Gait Problems in Cerebral Palsy*. London: MacKeith Press.

Baumann JU, Hanggi A. (1977) A method of gait analysis for daily orthopaedic practice. *Journal of Medical Engineering and Technology* **1**: 86–91.

Chung CY, Stout J, Gage JR. (1997) Rectus femoris transfer – gracilis versus sartorius. *Gait and Posture* **6**: 137–146.

du Plessis AJ. (2004) Mechanisms and manifestations of prenatal and perinatal brain injury. In: Gage JR (ed.) *The Treatment of Gait Problems in Cerebral Palsy*. London: MacKeith Press.

Gage JR. (1983) Gait analysis for decision-making in cerebral palsy. *Bulletin of the Hospital for Joint Diseases Orthopaedic Institute* **43**: 147–163.

Gage JR. (1991) *Gait Analysis in Cerebral Palsy*. London: MacKeith Press.

Gage JR. (ed.) (2004) *The Treatment of Gait Problems in Cerebral Palsy*. London: MacKeith Press.

Gage JR, Schwartz M. (2004) Pathological gait and lever-arm dysfunction. In: Gage JR (ed.) *The Treatment of Gait Problems in Cerebral Palsy*. London: MacKeith Press.

Gage JR, Perry J, Hicks RR *et al.* (1987) Rectus femoris transfer to improve knee function of children with cerebral palsy. *Developmental Medicine and Child Neurology* **29**: 159–166.

Graham HK, Aoki KR, Autti-Rämö I *et al.* (2000) Recommendations for the use of botulinum toxin type A in the management of cerebral palsy. *Gait and Posture* **11**: 67–79.

Lin C-J, Guo L-Y, Su F-C *et al.* (2000) Common abnormal kinetic patterns of the knee in gait in spastic diplegia of cerebral palsy. *Gait and Posture* **11**: 224–232.

Miller F, Cardoso Dias R, Lipton GE *et al.* (1997) The effect of rectus EMG patterns on the outcome of rectus femoris transfers. *Journal of Pediatric Orthopedics* **17**: 603–607.

Novacheck TF. (2004) Diplegia and quadriplegia. In: Gage JR (ed.) *The Treatment of Gait Problems in Cerebral Palsy*. London: MacKeith Press.

Olney SJ, Richards C. (1996). Hemiparetic gait following stroke. Part I: characteristics. *Gait and Posture* **4**: 136–148.

Õunpuu S. (2004) Patterns of gait pathology. In: Gage JR (ed.) *The Treatment of Gait Problems in Cerebral Palsy*. London: MacKeith Press.

Õunpuu S, Davis RB, DeLuca PA. (1996) Joint kinetics: methods, interpretation and treatment decision-making in children with cerebral palsy and myelomeningocele. *Gait and Posture* **4**: 62–78.

Peacock WJ. (2004) The pathophysiology of spasticity. In: Gage JR (ed.) *The Treatment of Gait Problems in Cerebral Palsy*. London: MacKeith Press.

Perry J. (1969) The mechanics of walking in hemiplegia. *Clinical Orthopaedics and Related Research* **63**: 23–31.

Perry J. (1987) Distal rectus femoris transfer. *Developmental Medicine and Child Neurology* **29**: 153–158.

Perry J. (1990) Pathologic gait. *American Academy of Orthopaedic Surgeons: Instructional Course Lectures* **39**: 325–331.

Perry J. (1992) *Gait Analysis: Normal and Pathological Function*. Thorofare, NJ: Slack Incorporated.

Richards CL, Olney SJ. (1996) Hemiparetic gait following stroke. Part II: recovery and physical therapy. *Gait and Posture* **4**: 149–162.

Rose GK. (1983) Clinical gait assessment: a personal view. *Journal of Medical Engineering and Technology* **7**: 273–279.

Schutte LM, Narayanan U, Stout JL *et al.* (2000) An index for quantifying deviations from normal gait. *Gait and Posture* **11**: 25–31.

Stout J, Koop S. (2004) Energy expenditure in cerebral palsy. In: Gage JR (ed.) *The Treatment of Gait Problems in Cerebral Palsy.* London: MacKeith Press.

Stout JL, Gage JR, Bruce R. (1994) Joint kinetic patterns in spastic hemiplegia (abstract). *Developmental Medicine and Child Neurology* **70**(Suppl): 8–9.

Sutherland DH. (1990) Gait analysis in neuromuscular diseases. *American Academy of Orthopaedic Surgeons: Instructional Course Lectures* **39**: 333–341.

Sutherland DH, Cooper L. (1978) The pathomechanics of progressive crouch gait in spastic diplegia. *Orthopedic Clinics of North America* **9**: 143–154.

Trost J. (2004) Physical assessment and observational gait analysis. In: Gage JR (ed.) *The Treatment of Gait Problems in Cerebral Palsy.* London: MacKeith Press.

Waters RL, Garland DE, Perry J *et al.* (1979) Stiff-legged gait in hemiplegia: surgical correction. *Journal of Bone and Joint Surgery* **61A**: 927–933.

Winters TF, Gage JR, Hicks R. (1987) Gait patterns in spastic hemiplegia in children and young adults. *Journal of Bone and Joint Surgery* **69A**: 437–441.

Gait analysis data on CD-ROM

7

This textbook is accompanied by a CD-ROM, which is designed to give the reader access to some 'real' gait data, both from a normal subject and from three individuals with cerebral palsy. The data were collected at Denver Children's Hospital, using the Vicon system. The multimedia presentation was prepared using the powerful 'Vicon Polygon' program. The CD-ROM includes 'Polygon Viewer', which is used to view reports made using the 'Polygon Authoring Tool'. Both Vicon and Polygon are products of Vicon Peak.

COMPUTER REQUIREMENTS

This CD will run on Windows only. To function properly, your computer should support at least an 800 × 600 pixel screen resolution, 256 colours, 128 MB RAM, and operate on Windows 2000 or above.

RUNNING THE CD

If the 'autorun' facility has been enabled on the computer, the Polygon Viewer program should start automatically after the CD-ROM has been inserted. If this does not happen, there are two possible ways to start the program.

1. Use Windows Explorer to navigate to the CD drive (usually D:) and double-click on 'Startup.exe'.

2. Click on the 'Start' icon, select 'Run...', type in 'D:Startup' (without spaces, and without the quotation marks), and press the Enter key. If the CD drive is not D:, substitute the appropriate drive letter in the command.

CONTENTS OF THE CD

1. How to use the Polygon Viewer (repeated below)
2. A normal adult female subject walking
3. A 16-year-old male with a crouch gait due to spastic diplegia cerebral palsy
4. An 8-year-old male with equinus on both sides due to spastic diplegia cerebral palsy
5. A 9-year-old female with a stiff left knee due to left hemiplegia cerebral palsy

HOW TO USE THE POLYGON VIEWER (BY DR CHRIS KIRTLEY)

The workspace allows you to see four types of display, known as 'panes':

1. a movie of the subject walking
2. a workspace with 3D animation (skeleton)
3. a number of pages of text
4. a number of graphs.

How to manipulate the skeleton

You can turn the skeleton around by left-dragging the mouse. You can also zoom in or out by right-dragging the mouse up or down. Finally you can move the skeleton up and down or side to side by clicking and holding both mouse buttons. Have a try, and you'll soon get the hang of it!

The force vectors (yellow) can be turned off by right-clicking anywhere on the display and selecting 'Force Vectors' in the 'Hide Objects' menu.

Controlling the movie and workspace: the time bar

The time bar (at the bottom of the screen) has two main parts. The left part has six buttons, a slider and two number displays, and works more or less like a video recorder or CD player. The time ruler shows the current position in the gait cycle, indicated by a cursor (an open downward-directed pointer). You can move the animation and movie by dragging this cursor to the left or right using the left mouse button. If you miss the cursor and left-drag, you'll scroll the whole time bar ruler left or right. If you right-drag, you will alter the scale on the time bar. The default setting can be restored by double-clicking the ruler with the left mouse button, or right-clicking and selecting 'Full Size'.

The buttons on the left-hand side of the time bar are fairly intuitive – click the leftmost button to play the animation and movie backwards, the one next to it to play forwards. Also note that when you press either of the 'play' buttons, it changes to a 'stop' button – you start motion by pressing the button once and stop it by pressing it again. The two upper right buttons are for stepping forwards and backwards one frame at the time. The two buttons below also step forwards and backwards but instead of stepping one frame at a time, they step to the next or previous event or, if there are none, to the start or end of the animation. The events are the little symbols under the time ruler and define each gait cycle by initial contact (diamond) and toe off (upward arrow) of that foot.

The slider (bottom left-hand corner) controls the replay speed. The replay speed is a number between 0.1 and 2.0 and determines the speed of the animations relative to real time. 1.0 is real time, 2.0 is twice as fast and 0.1 is one-tenth of real time.

Right-clicking the time bar lets you select or de-select 'Toggle Replay Loop'. When selected, there are two little cursors at either end of the current range of the animation (if you can't see them it's probably because you've zoomed or moved the ruler; double-click and everything should be OK). These let you watch only part of the trial. You can move them by left-dragging and you will see that when you subsequently hit 'play', the motion will wrap around when the current time cursor hits either of the replay loop cursors. This is very useful if you repeatedly want to study a little subsection of the motion, for example an interesting part of the gait cycle.

The graph pane

This display shows the knee angle in the sagittal (flexion/extension), transverse (rotation) and frontal (ab/adduction = valgus/varus) planes. The left side is red and the right side green – port and starboard, as in the navigation lights of ships! Double-clicking one of the graphs will show it by itself; the other graphs are then available by clicking the 'tabs' at the top of the display. Double-clicking a single graph returns to the 'thumbnail' (several graphs) display.

In some of the graphs the normal pattern for that age is shown in pale gray.

As usual, the horizontal axis is percent of the gait cycle, with stance phase to the left, and a vertical line to indicate the start of swing phase.

The cursor in the time bar determines which cycles are shown; moving the cursor from range 1 on the left side to range 2 changes the left-side graph slightly. The position of the cursor is shown by a green (right) or red (left) line, although this is not always visible in the thumbnail view, if the graphs are too small.

You can also perform other manipulations on the graphs, such as zooming in and out or selecting particular ranges, by right-clicking on different graph elements, and choosing items from the menu.

Moving and removing panes

If you want to move text, movie, animation or graphs on the screen you can use the 'Move Pane' button (two gray boxes, connected by a red arrow). Click the button, then click in the pane you want to move and click again where you want to put it. If you want to completely get rid of a pane, use the 'Remove Pane' button next to it (a gray box containing a red 'X').

The size of panes may be altered by dragging their borders, using the left mouse button.

Notes

1. The bars representing normal EMG activity are from Wootten ME, Kadaba MP, Cochran GV. (1990) Dynamic electromyography. II. Normal patterns during gait. *Journal of Orthopaedic Research* **8**: 259–265. However, EMG patterns are very variable and these bars only represent a 'typical' pattern.
2. The video data and the walking skeleton sometimes don't synchronize until the loop has been played once or twice. Where two walking skeletons are shown, the video is synchronized to the 'abnormal' one.

Acknowledgments

Sincere thanks are given to the following, who have made this CD possible.
1. Nancy Denniston, from the Denver Children's Hospital, for a great deal of hard work in preparing the majority of this CD. Thanks are also due to her colleagues, including Dr James Carollo and Kristin Ness.
2. Vicon Peak for allowing Nancy Denniston and the author of this book to use version 3.1 of the Vicon Polygon Authoring Tool software. Vicon Peak may be found on the Internet at www.vicon.com/, or contacted by email at sales@vicon.com. Their postal address, telephone and fax numbers are as follows:
Head Office: Vicon Peak, 14 Minns Business Park, West Way, Oxford OX2 0JB, UK.
Tel: +44 (0) 1865 261800 Fax: +44 (0) 1865 240527
In USA: Vicon Peak, 9 Spectrum Pointe Drive, Lake Forest, CA 92630. Tel: (949) 472 9140 Fax: (949) 472 9136
Vicon Peak, 7388 S. Revere Parkway Suite 901, Centennial, CO 80112. Tel: (303) 799 8686 Fax: (303) 799 8690

Appendix

I

Approximate range (95% limits) for general gait parameters in free-speed walking by normal FEMALE subjects of different ages

Age (years)	Cadence (steps/min)	Cycle time (s)	Stride length (m)	Speed (m/s)
13–14	103–150	0.80–1.17	0.99–1.55	0.90–1.62
15–17	100–144	0.83–1.20	1.03–1.57	0.92–1.64
18–49	98–138	0.87–1.22	1.06–1.58	0.94–1.66
50–64	97–137	0.88–1.24	1.04–1.56	0.91–1.63
65–80	96–136	0.88–1.25	0.94–1.46	0.80–1.52

Approximate range (95% limits) for general gait parameters in free-speed walking by normal MALE subjects of different ages

Age (years)	Cadence (steps/min)	Cycle time (s)	Stride length (m)	Speed (m/s)
13–14	100–149	0.81–1.20	1.06–1.64	0.95–1.67
15–17	96–142	0.85–1.25	1.15–1.75	1.03–1.75
18–49	91–135	0.89–1.32	1.25–1.85	1.10–1.82
50–64	82–126	0.95–1.46	1.22–1.82	0.96–1.68
65–80	81–125	0.96 –1.48	1.11–1.71	0.81–1.61

Approximate range (95% limits) for general gait parameters in free-speed walking by normal CHILDREN of different ages. (Ages one to seven based on reference Sutherland *et al.*, 1988)

Age (years)	Cadence (steps/min)	Cycle time (s)	Stride length (m)	Speed (m/s)
1	127–223	0.54–0.94	0.29–0.58	0.32–0.96
1.5	126–212	0.57–0.95	0.33–0.66	0.39–1.03
2	125–201	0.60–0.96	0.37–0.73	0.45–1.09
2.5	124–190	0.63–0.97	0.42–0.81	0.52–1.16
3	123–188	0.64–0.98	0.46–0.89	0.58–1.22
3.5	122–186	0.65–0.98	0.50–0.96	0.65–1.29
4	121–184	0.65–0.99	0.54–1.04	0.67–1.32
5	119–180	0.67–1.01	0.59–1.10	0.71–1.37
6	117–176	0.68–1.03	0.64–1.16	0.75–1.43
7	115–172	0.70–1.04	0.69–1.22	0.80–1.48
8	113–169	0.71–1.06	0.75–1.30	0.82–1.50
9	111–166	0.72–1.08	0.82–1.37	0.83–1.53
10	109–162	0.74–1.10	0.88–1.45	0.85–1.55
11	107–159	0.75–1.12	0.92–1.49	0.86–1.57
12	105–156	0.77–1.14	0.96–1.54	0.88–1.60

Appendix

2

For each variable, the Système International d'Unités (SI) uses a fundamental unit and a series of multiples and submultiples, in steps of 10^3, as follows:

pico (p) 10^{-12} kilo (k) 10^3
nano (n) 10^{-9} mega (M) 10^6
micro (µ) 10^{-6} giga (G) 10^9
milli (m) 10^{-3} tera (T) 10^{12}

Length

SI units: millimeter (mm), meter (m), kilometer (km)
Other units: inch (in), foot (ft), mile (mi)

1 mm = 0.039370 in
1 m = 1000 mm = 39.370 in = 3.2808 ft
1 km = 1000 m = 0.62137 mi

Area

SI unit: square millimeter (mm^2), square meter (m^2)
Other units: square inch (in^2), square foot (ft^2)

$1 \ mm^2 = 0.0015500 \ in^2$
$1 \ m^2 = 10^6 \ mm^2 = 10.764 \ ft^2$

Volume

SI units: cubic millimeter (mm^3), cubic meter (m^3)
Other units: milliliter (ml), liter (l), cubic inch (in^3), cubic foot (ft^3), fluid ounce (fl oz), gallon (gal)

1 ml = 1000 mm^3 = 0.061024 in^3
1 l = 1000 ml = 35.195 fl oz (UK) = 33.814 fl oz (US)
1 m^3 = 1000 l = 219.97 gal (UK) = 264.17 gal (US) = 35.315 ft^3

Linear velocity

SI unit: meter per second (m/s or m s^{-1})
Other units: feet per second (ft/s or ft s^{-1}), kilometers per hour (kph), miles per hour (mph)

1 m/s = 3.2808 ft/s = 3.6000 kph = 2.2369 mph

Linear acceleration

SI unit: meter per second per second (m/s^2 or m s^{-2})
Other units: feet per second per second (ft/s^2 or ft s^{-2})

1 m/s^2 = 3.2808 ft/s^2

Acceleration due to gravity

g = 9.80665 m/s^{-2} = 32.174 ft s^{-2}

Mass

SI units: gram (g), kilogram (kg)
Other units: ounce (oz), pound (lb), slug

1 g = 0.035274 oz
1 kg = 1000 g = 2.2046 lb = 0.068522 slug

Force

SI unit: newton (N) (equivalent to kg·m/s^2)
Other units: dyne (dyn), kilogram force (kg f), kilopond (kp) - identical to kilogram force, pound force (lb f), poundal (pdl)

$1 \text{ N} = 10^5 \text{ dyn} = 0.10197 \text{ kg f} = 0.22481 \text{ lb f} = 7.2330 \text{ pdl}$

Pressure and stress

SI units: pascal (Pa), kilopascal (kPa), megapascal (MPa)
Other units: bar, millimeter of mercury (mmHg), inch of water (in H$_2$O), physical atmosphere (atm), pound force per square inch (psi), kilogram force per square centimeter (kg f/cm^2)

$1 \text{ Pa} = 1 \text{ N m}^{-2} = 10^{-5} \text{ bar}$
$1 \text{ kPa} = 1000 \text{ Pa} = 4.0146 \text{ in H}_2\text{O} = 7.5006 \text{ mmHg}$
$1 \text{ MPa} = 1000 \text{ kPa} = 9.8692 \text{ atm} = 145.04 \text{ psi} = 10.197 \text{ kg f/cm}^2$

Energy

SI units: joule (J), kilojoule (kJ), megajoule (MJ)
Other units: erg, 15° calorie, 15° kilocalorie (kcal$_{15}$) – identical to Calorie, used in dietary calculations, British thermal unit (Btu), kilowatt hour (kWh)

$1 \text{ J} = 10^7 \text{ erg} = 0.23892 \text{ cal}_{15}$
$1 \text{ kJ} = 1000 \text{ J} = 0.23892 \text{ kcal}_{15} = 0.94781 \text{ Btu}$
$1 \text{ MJ} = 1000 \text{ kJ} = 0.27778 \text{ kWh}$

Power

SI units: watt (W), kilowatt (kW)
Other unit: horsepower (hp)

$1 \text{ W} = 1 \text{ J s}^{-1}$
$1 \text{ kW} = 1.3410 \text{ hp}$

Plane angle

SI unit: radian (rad)
Other unit: degree (°)

$180° = \pi$ rad
1 rad $= 180/\pi = 57.296°$
$1° = 0.017453$ rad

Appendix

3

SOURCES OF FURTHER INFORMATION

Journal articles

Papers in the scientific journals constitute the major repository for knowledge on any scientific subject, including gait analysis. A number of key papers are cited as references in this book. A computer search of the Medline database, using suitable keywords, will uncover many more. As well as its availability through research libraries, it is also possible to access Medline on the Internet, through the PubMed service (www.ncbi.nlm.nih.gov/PubMed/).

Papers on gait analysis are most frequently found in the following journals, although a large number of other journals also contain occasional papers on the subject:

Clinical Biomechanics
Clinical Orthopaedics and Related Research
Gait and Posture
Journal of Biomechanics
Journal of Biomedical Engineering
Journal of Bone and Joint Surgery
Physical Therapy

Learned societies

There are a number of learned societies which focus on gait analysis and related subjects, including the Gait and Clinical Movement Analysis Society

229

(GCMAS), the International Society for Postural and Gait Research (ISPG), the European Society of Movement Analysis in Adults and Children (ESMAC), and the Società Italiana di Analisi del Movimento in Clinica (SIAMOC). An even greater number of societies include gait analysis among their interests, including the International Society of Biomechanics (ISB) and the various national and regional societies of biomechanics. Up-to-date information on these societies will be found on the Internet (see below).

Conferences and conference proceedings

The most up-to-date information on gait analysis research will always be found in the oral and poster presentations at relevant conferences. The conferences with the highest content of gait analysis research are those run by the organizations listed in the preceding section. Details of forthcoming conferences will be found in the calendar sections of some of the journals, and on the Internet (see below). Many conferences publish books of proceedings or abstracts, which are available for purchase. Few libraries have these books and it is usually necessary to contact the conference organizers to obtain them. Exceptions to this are the GCMAS, ESMAC and SIAMOC meetings, the abstracts from which are published in the journal *Gait and Posture*.

Textbooks

Each of the chapters in this book ends in a bibliography, which lists some major texts, providing further information on the topics covered by the chapter.

Videotapes

A number of individuals and institutions have developed videotapes as learning aids for gait analysis. Those the author is aware of are as follows.

Physical examination of the musculoskeletal system, program 9: gait, by Larry B. Conochie

American Academy of Orthopedic Surgeons
222 South Prospect Avenue
Park Ridge, Illinois 60068, USA

Normal development of walking, by Janet L. Hale
Therapy Skill Builders
3830 E. Bellevue
P.O. Box 42050
Tucson, Arizona 85733, USA

Observation of human gait (in 3 parts)
Health Sciences Media Services 0J1 WMC
University of Alberta
Edmonton, Alberta T6G 2R7, Canada

1. Normal walking
2. Principles of pathologic gait in cerebral palsy
Gillette Children's Hospital
200 East University Avenue
St Paul, Minnesota 55101, USA
Phone: +1-612-291-2848

Several other videos on gait are available from:
Los Amigos Research and Education Institute, Inc.
P.O. Box 3500
12841 Dahlia St., Bldg. #306
Downey, California 90242, USA

Computer programs

The following computer programs are also likely to be useful for learning about gait and gait analysis

GaitCD (CD-ROM, for IBM-PC running Windows 95 or later)
Christopher L. Vaughan (1999) ISBN 0 620 23561 6.
Kiboho Publishers
P.O. Box 769
Howard Place
Western Cape 7450
South Africa

Normal walking and *Principles of pathologic gait in cerebral palsy* (CD-ROM, for IBM-PC or Macintosh)
Gillette Children's Hospital (address in 'Videotapes' above)

BioWare force platform analysis software (for IBM-PC)
Kistler Instrumente AG Winterthur
P.O. Box 304
CH-8408 Winterthur
Switzerland

The Internet

The Internet is changing extremely rapidly. The information below is current at the time of publication, but may be somewhat out of date by the time you read this!

Probably the most useful resource is the Clinical Gait Analysis website (http://guardian.curtin.edu.au/cga/).

A great deal of information on gait analysis can also be found on the biomechanics 'list', known as BIOMCH-L (http://isb.ri.ccf.org/biomch-l/index.html/).

Some information about gait analysis is included in the Kinesiology and Biomechanics Teacher's Information Service (www.usfca.edu/ess/tis/).

Many other Internet sites contain information relevant to gait analysis, which can be found by entering suitable keywords into a search engine, such as Google. Further information is available from the many books about the Internet or from the providers of the on-line services.

Glossary

Abduction – movement of a limb away from the midline, in the frontal plane.

Adduction – movement of a limb towards the midline, in the frontal plane.

Afferent – nerves or nerve impulses reaching the central nervous system from peripheral parts of the body.

Aiming – walking in an unnatural way, so that the foot will land in a particular position, e.g. on a force platform.

Anatomical position – used for anatomical descriptions: standing upright, with the feet together, the arms by the sides and the palms forward.

Ankylosis – destruction of a joint, either by surgery or disease, resulting in a total loss of movement.

Anoxia – a complete lack of oxygen in part of the body, e.g. the brain.

Antagonists – muscles with opposing actions, e.g. flexion *versus* extension.

Anterior – to the front of the body (in the anatomical position).

Anteversion – a rotation of part of the body (e.g. the upper femur) so that it faces anteriorly.

Ataxia – loss of coordination, due to disease of the central nervous system.

Athetosis – disorder of the central nervous system, resulting in continual uncoordinated movements of the limbs.

Atrophy – loss of bulk, especially of a muscle.

Baclofen – a drug used to reduce muscle tone.

Basal gangia – neurological centers deep within the cerebral cortex, which plan and supervise limb movements.

Biarticular muscle – a muscle which crosses two joints between its origin and insertion.

Biofeedback – allowing a person to see how well they are performing a task, so that they can make immediate improvements.

Botulinum toxin ('Botox') – used by injection to paralyze muscles; the effects generally last about 3 months.

Bunion – see *hallux valgus*.

Butterfly diagram – method of displaying ground reaction force data.

Cadence – the number of steps (not strides) in a given time, usually 1 minute.

Calcaneus deformity – a deformity in which the forefoot points upwards, so that typically only the heel contacts the ground.

Calliper – orthosis (q.v.) fitted around one or both legs, to compensate for weakness or paralysis; also spelled caliper.

Caudad – towards the 'tail'; equivalent of inferior.

Center of gravity – in mechanical calculations, the point within an object at which it can be assumed that the mass of the object is concentrated.

Center of pressure – the point beneath the foot through which it can be assumed that the ground reaction force is passing.

Central pattern generator – networks of neurons (q.v.) in the brain and spinal cord, which act together to generate repetitive motions, such as walking.

Cephalad – towards the head; equivalent of superior.

Cerebellar ataxia – ataxia (q.v.) due to disease of the cerebellum.

Cerebral palsy (CP) – neurological disorder with spasticity (q.v.) and incoordination, usually caused by brain damage before birth.

Cerebrovascular accident (CVA) – brain damage due to blood clot or hemorrhage; also known as stroke.

Clonus – jerky contraction of a muscle, usually due to spasticity (q.v.).

Co-contraction – when two diferent muscles contract at the same time.

Cognitive – relating to the ability to think normally.

Concentric contraction – muscle contraction in which the muscle gets shorter as it develops tension.

Congenital dislocation of hip (CDH) – condition present at birth in which the head of femur is not properly contained in the acetabulum.

Contracture – reduction in the range of motion of a joint, due to restriction by inelastic connective tissue.

Coronal plane – see *frontal plane*.

Couple – two parallel forces acting in opposite directions, which combine to produce a moment (q.v.).

Coupled movements – see *coupling*.

Coupling – due to the alignment of a joint, movement in one direction automatically produces movement in another direction.

Coxa valga – abnormal angulation of the upper end of the femur, making the femoral neck too vertical.

Coxa vara – abnormal angulation of the upper end of the femur, making the femoral neck too horizontal.

Cycle time – the time taken to complete a single gait cycle.

Deep – far from the surface.

Derotation osteotomy – operation in which a long bone is cut through and held in a partially rotated position while it heals.

Determinants of gait – six strategies used to minimize energy consumption in normal gait.

Diabetes – disease in which control of blood sugar is imperfect, through lack of, or abnormal response to, the hormone insulin.

Diabetic neuropathy – loss of function of peripheral nerves, especially sensory nerves in the feet, due to diabetes (q.v.).

Diplegia – paralysis of both arms or both legs.

Distal – away from the rest of the body.

Dorsal – the posterior surface.

Dorsal rhizotomy – selective cutting of some of the sensory fibers in the posterior (dorsal) root of a number of spinal nerves. Used to reduce spasticity, by interfering with the stretch reflex.

Dorsiflexion – movement of the foot towards the knee.

Dorsum – the back of the hand, or the upper surface of the foot.

Double pendulum – a structure which is suspended at its top end, but jointed in the middle. It can swing like a pendulum about both joints.

Double support – period in the gait cycle in which both feet are on the ground, one in loading response and one in pre-swing.

Dyskinesia – abnormal limb movements, such as incoordination or waving limbs around, caused by brain damage.

Eccentric contraction – muscle contraction in which the external force overpowers the muscle so that it gets longer.

Efferent – nerves or nerve impulses leaving the central nervous system, directed towards peripheral parts of the body.

Electrogoniometer – device which fixes across a joint and puts out a continuous electrical signal describing joint angle.

Electromyogram (EMG) – recording of the electrical activity of a muscle.

Embolism – blockage of an artery, cutting off the blood supply, typically by a blood clot.

Engram – a method of performing a particular movement, learned by repetition.

Equinovarus – a foot deformity in which the foot points downwards and medially, ground contact being typically by the lateral border of the forefoot.

Equinus – a foot deformity in which the foot points downwards, ground contact being typically by the forefoot.

Evert, eversion – internal rotation about the long axis of the foot.

Extension – sagittal plane movement at a joint, the distal segment usually moving posteriorly (anteriorly at the knee).

External moment – moment applied from outside, as by an external force which is attempting to flex or extend a joint.

External rotation – rotation of a limb about its long axis, the anterior surface moving laterally.

Extrapyramidal system – areas of the brain and spinal cord providing coordination and control, as opposed to direct activation of muscles.

Feet adjacent – event in the swing phase of the gait cycle when the foot of the swinging leg passes the supporting foot.

Flexion – sagittal plane movement at a joint, the distal segment usually moving anteriorly (posteriorly at the knee).

Flexion contracture – deformity in which contraction of soft tissues prevents a joint from extending fully.

Foot flat – point in the stance phase of the gait cycle at which the forefoot contacts the ground, when initial contact has been made by the heel.

Foot slap – abrupt and audible lowering of the foot following initial contact (q.v.).

Footstrike – see *initial contact*.

Force platform, forceplate – common piece of gait analysis equipment, for measuring the ground reaction force (q.v.).

Forefoot – the five metatarsal bones and the toes.

Frontal plane – divides a body part into front and back portions.

Gait – the manner or style of walking.

Gait cycle – the time interval between two successive occurrences of one of the repetitive events of walking (usually initial contact on one side).

Ground reaction force – the upward force applied by the ground to the foot, in response to the downward force applied by the foot to the ground. Commonly measured by force platforms.

Hallux – the big toe or great toe.

Hallux valgus – deformity affecting the big toe,in which the metatarsophalangeal joint is in valgus; also known as bunion.

Hansen's disease – bacterial infection causing progressive destruction of nerves and sensory loss; also known as leprosy.

Heel rise – event in the stance phase of the gait cycle at which the heel lifts away from the supporting surface.

Heelstrike – a distinct impact between the heel and the ground at initial contact.

Hemiparesis – partial paralysis affecting one side of the body.

Hemiplegia – complete paralysis affecting one side of the body, usually due to brain disease or injury.

Hemorrhage – abnormal bleeding. Hemorrhage into the brain is a common cause of brain damage.

High tibial osteotomy – operation to change the alignment of the upper tibia, to alter the direction of forces acting on the knee.

Hindfoot – two bones in the foot: talus and calcaneus.

Horizontal plane - see *transverse plane*.

Hypoxia – a partial lack of oxygen in part of the body, e.g. the brain.

Inferior – lower down the body (in the anatomical position).

Initial contact – event in the gait cycle when first contact is made between the foot and ground; made by the heel in normal gait. Marks the transition from swing phase to stance phase.

Initial swing – period in the swing phase of the gait cycle between toe off and feet adjacent.

Internal moment – moment generated by muscles and/or ligaments in the vicinity of a joint.

Internal rotation – rotation of a limb about its long axis, the anterior surface moving medially.

Intrafusal – a specialized muscle fiber within a muscle spindle (q.v.).

Intrathecal – injection into the fluid surrounding the spinal cord.

Invert, inversion – external rotation about the long axis of the foot.

Isometric contraction – muscle contraction in which a muscle develops tension but remains the same length.

Lateral – away from the midline of the body.

Lateral rotation – see *external rotation*.

Lever arm – the perpendicular distance between a force and the axis of rotation, when generating a moment (q.v.).

Line of gravity – a vertical line downwards from the center of gravity (q.v.).

Line of progression – straight line corresponding to the average path taken by the body in walking.

Loading response – period in the stance phase of the gait cycle between initial contact and opposite toe off.

Lordosis – forward curvature of the spine, causing concavity of the lumbar region of the back.

Lower motor neuron – nerve fiber producing muscular contraction, running from the spinal cord to the muscle.

Marker – an object fixed to a point on the skin, so that it is visible to an optical measurement system. Typically a small sphere covered in reflective tape.

Medial – towards the midline of the body.

Medial rotation – see *internal rotation*.

Median plane – the midline sagittal plane, which divides the whole body into right and left halves.

Metatarsalgia – severe pain beneath the metatarsal heads, typically caused by nerve compression.

Midfoot – five tarsal bones: navicular, cuboid and the medial, intermediate and lateral cuneiforms.

Mid-stance – period in the stance phase of the gait cycle between opposite toe off and heel rise.

Mid-swing – period in the swing phase of the gait cycle between feet adjacent and tibia vertical.

Moment, moment of force – a turning effect; typically a force being applied in such a way that it causes a rotation.

Moment arm – see *lever arm*.

Monarticular muscle – a muscle which only crosses one joint between its origin and insertion.

Multiple sclerosis – progressive neurological disease, caused by a patchy loss of myelin from neurons in brain and spinal cord.

Muscle spindle – sense organ embedded within a muscle, to monitor muscle tension. It contains intrafusal muscle fibers (q.v.) which contract to adjust its sensitivity.

Muscular dystrophy – progressive wasting disease affecting muscles, usually hereditary.

Neonatal jaundice – high levels of bilirubin in the blood of a newborn child, from red cells destroyed by antibodies from the mother. It produces yellowing of the skin, and brain damage if severe.

Noise – random errors which affect any form of measurement.

Opposite initial contact – event in the stance phase of the gait cycle when the other foot makes initial contact with the ground; occurs at around 50% of the cycle in normal gait.

Opposite toe off – event in the stance phase of the gait cycle when the other foot is leaving the ground. Generally close in time to foot flat (q.v.).

Oral – taken by mouth.

Orthosis – an external support for some part of the body; also known as brace.

Osteo-arthritis – degenerative disease affecting the joints, with pain, stiffness and deformity.

Osteotomy – surgical operation involving cutting through a bone. An abnormally rotated bone may be cut through, rotated and allowed to heal in the new position.

Paralysis – loss of the ability to voluntarily contract a muscle.

Paraplegia – complete paralysis of the legs, usually due to disease or injury of the spinal cord.

Paresis – partial paralysis.

Parkinsonism – progressive degenerative neurological condition, involving tremor and weakness; also known as Parkinson's disease.

Patella alta – deformity in which the patella is more proximal than usual, generally through stretching of the patellar tendon.

Patterned responses, primitive reflexes – movement patterns which are 'pre-programmed' into the nervous system, e.g. flexor withdrawal, in which the flexor muscles contract to withdraw the foot from a painful stimulus.

Perineum – the area of skin around the anus and genitalia.

Peripheral nerves – nerves which originate in the spinal cord, as opposed to cranial nerves, which originate in the brain.

Peripheral neuropathy – loss of function due to degeneration of the nerves of the hands and feet.

Physiological cost index (PCI) – method of estimating relative energy consumption using the heart rate.

Plane of progression – a flat vertical plane following the average path taken by the body in walking.

Plantarflexion – movement of the foot away from the knee.

Poliomyelitis – virus disease causing destruction of lower motor neurons, with muscle atrophy and paralysis.

Posterior – to the back of the body (in the anatomical position).

Prematurity – birth before full gestation. Typically, birth earlier than 36 weeks gestation carries an increased risk to the child.

Pressure sore – ulcer (q.v.) forming on an area of skin exposed to sufficient pressure to cut off the blood supply.

Pre-swing – period in the stance phase of the gait cycle between opposite initial contact and toe off.

Pronation – forearm: internal rotation; foot: a combination of eversion, dorsiflexion and forefoot abduction.

Proprioception – unconscious feedback on joint position, force in ligaments and tendons, etc.

Prosthetic joint – an artificial joint, implanted in place of the natural joint.

Prosthetic limb – an artificial limb, usually fixed onto a stump following amputation.

Proximal – towards the rest of the body.

Push off – see *pre-swing*.

Quadriplegia – paralysis of both arms and both legs; also known as tetraplegia.

Rheumatoid arthritis – painful inflammation of the joints, caused by a connective tissue disease.

Rhizotomy – see *dorsal rhizotomy*.

Rockers – the three mechanisms used to move the tibia forward while the foot is on the ground.

Sagittal plane – divides part of the body into right and left portions.

Selective dorsal rhizotomy – see *dorsal rhizotomy*.

Single support – period during the gait cycle in which only one foot is in contact with the ground; corresponds to swing phase on the other side.

Slipped femoral epiphysis – hip disease involving displacement of the articular surface of the femoral head, typically in teenagers.

Spastic diplegia – variety of cerebral palsy (q.v.) in which the two lower limbs are affected more than the upper limbs.

Spastic hemiplegia – variety of cerebral palsy (q.v.) in which the arm and leg on one side are affected more than the arm and leg on the other side.

Spastic triplegia – variety of cerebral palsy (q.v.) in which the two lower limbs and one arm are principally affected.

Spasticity – involuntary resistance of muscles to being stretched.

Spina bifida – incomplete development of the vertebrae, resulting in damage to the associated spinal cord.

Stance phase – that part of the gait cycle for one side in which the foot is on the ground.

Stance time – the duration of the stance phase, between initial contact and toe off.

Step – the advancement of a single foot.

Step length – the distance one foot moves ahead of the other foot during the gait cycle.

Step-to, step-through – gait patterns used when walking with crutches.

Stride – the advancement of both feet (one step by each side).

Stride length – the distance either foot moves forward during the gait cycle.

Stroke – see *cerebrovascular accident*.

Subcutaneous – beneath the skin.

Subluxation – partial dislocation of a joint, the joint surfaces being able to move in and out of the correct alignment.

Superficial – close to the surface.

Superior – higher up the body (in the anatomical position).

Supination – forearm: external rotation; foot: inversion, plantarflexion and forefoot adduction.

Swing phase – that part of the gait cycle for one side in which the foot is off the ground, moving through the air.

Swing time – the duration of the swing phase, between toe off and initial contact.

Syndrome – a medical condition in which a number of different signs or symptoms typically occur.

Tabes dorsalis – loss of sensation and proprioception, due to effect of syphilis on the sensory pathways of the spinal cord.

Tenotomy – surgical cutting of a tendon, either to free it completely or to lengthen or shorten it.

Terminal stance – period in the stance phase of the gait cycle between heel rise and opposite initial contact.

Terminal swing – period in the swing phase of the gait cycle between tibia vertical and the next initial contact.

Tetraparesis – partial paralysis affecting all four limbs.

Tetraplegia – see *quadriplegia*.

Tibia vertical – event in the swing phase of gait in which the tibia passes through the vertical in moving from behind the body to in front of it.

Toe drag – failure to clear the ground with the toes during the swing phase of gait.

Toe in – the angle between the foot and the line of progression, when the toes are inclined medially.

Toe off – event in the gait cycle when the foot (generally the toe) leaves the ground. Marks the transition from the stance phase to the swing phase.

Toe out – the angle between the foot and the line of progression, when the toes are inclined laterally.

Toestrike – making initial contact (q.v.) with the toes, rather than the heel or flat foot.

Tone – the amount by which a muscle resists attempts to stretch it: high tone is present in spasticity (q.v.).

Torque – see *moment*.

Torsion – twisting. Often applied to a long bone (e.g. the femur) in which a 'twist' is present between the proximal and distal ends.

Transection – cutting through completely (applied to spinal cord).

Transfemoral amputation – amputation of a leg between the hip and knee joints.

Transtibial amputation – amputation of a leg between the knee and ankle joints.

Transverse plane – divides a body part into upper and lower portions.

Ulcer – loss of covering skin or epithelium.

Upper motor neuron – nerve fiber producing muscular contraction, running from the brain to the spinal cord, where it connects with lower motor neurons.

Valgus – joint angulation, with the distal segment sloping away from the midline.

Varus – joint angulation, with the distal segment sloping towards the midline.

Vaulting – gait abnormality in which the subject goes up on tiptoe during the stance phase of one leg, to increase the ground clearance of the other foot.

Ventral – the anterior surface.

Walking base – the side-to-side distance between the paths taken by the two feet.

Index

A

A band, 25
Abduction, 3
Abductor digiti minimi, 15
Abductor hallucis, 15
Abnormal gait, 101
  anterior trunk bending, 107-8,
    108, 114, 116, 129
  causes, 101, 102
    compensatory, 103
  clinical decision making, 179-80
  clinical diagnosis, 180, *181*, 185
  dorsiflexion control inadequacy,
    117
  foot contact abnormality, 117-18
  foot rotation abnormality, 119,
    122
  foot slap, 117
  functional leg length discrepancy,
    109-10, 116, 117, 198
    circumduction, 109, *111*, 111,
      113, 205
    hip hiking, 109, 111, *112*, 113
    steppage, 109, 111-12, *112*,
      113
  vaulting, 109, 112-13, *113*
  habit patterns, 185
  head/neck attitude/movement
    abnormality, 122
  hip rotation abnormality, 113-14
  knee flexion excess, *116*, 116-17
  knee hyperextension, 114-16, *115*
  lateral trunk bending, 103-7, *105*
  lever arm disease/deficiency, 119
  lumbar lordosis increase, 109, *110*
  movement abnormalities, 122
  posterior trunk bending, 108, *109*
  psychogenic causes, 185
  push off insufficiency, 120
  rapid fatigue, 122
  rhythmic disturbances, 121

  spastic hemiplegia, 197-8
  specific patterns, 102-22
  terminology, 102
  toe drag, 117
  upper limb attitude/movement
    abnormality, 122
  visual analysis, *138*, 138
    walkway length, 139
  walking base abnormality, 120-1
  see also Pathological gait
Above knee (transfemoral, AK)
    amputation, 129
  amputee gait, 129, *131*
  prosthesis design, 129-30
  knee mechanism, 130
Acceleration, 40, 41
  angular, 41
  kinematic measurements, 167
Accelerometers, 159-60, 167
  motion measurement, 160
  transients measurement, 159
Acetabulum, 5, 8
Acetylcholine, 27
Achilles tendon, 14
  insufficient push off, 120
  lengthening
    excessive, 201, 209
    spastic hemiplegia, 198
Actin, 25, *26*, 27
Action potential, 23
  muscle contraction stimulation, 27
  propagation, 23-4, *24*
  saltatory conduction, 24
Active insufficiency, 27
Active (internal) moment, 38
Active marker kinematic systems,
    172
Adduction, 3
Adductor brevis, 12
Adductor hallucis, 15
Adductor longus, 12, 72, 74, 76

Adductor magnus, 12
Adenosine triphosphate (ATP), 27,
    43
Aerobic metabolism, 27
Afferent neurons, 16, 22
Age-related changes, 47, 50, 96-8
  see also Elderly people
Agonist, 28
Amputation, 129
  above knee, 129-30, *131*
  ankle level, 129, 131, *132*, 133
  below knee, 129, 131-3, *132*
  femur/prosthetic limb mechanical
    coupling, 129
Amputee gait, 129-33, 187
  above knee amputation, 129, *131*
  ankle-level amputation, 131, *132*,
    133
  below knee amputation, 131-3,
    132
Anaerobic metabolism, 27
Analog-to-digital converter, 161, 164
Anatomical position, *2*, 2
Anatomy, 1-19
  bones, 5-8, *6*
  joints, 8-11
  ligaments, 8-11
  muscles, 11-15
  peripheral nerves, 18-19
  spinal cord, 15-18, *16*
  spinal nerves, 15-18
  tendons, 11-12
  terminology, 2-3
Angle-angle diagram (cyclogram),
    149, 149
Angular acceleration, 41
Angular momentum, 42
Angular velocity, 41
  kinematic measurements, 167
Ankle, *6*, 6, 9
  cerebral palsy, 205, *208*, 208

Ankle, (cont'd)
  determinants of gait, 91, 91
  feet adjacent, 77-8
  heel rise, 72, 73
  immobility, 116
  initial contact, 66
  ligaments, 10
  loading response, 67
  mid-stance, 70, 71
  moments, 67, 69, 71, 73, 74, 75, 76, 180
  movements, 4, 10
    children, 95
    elderly people, 98
    gait cycle, 63
    see also Coupled ankle/foot motion
  muscles, 14-15
  opposite initial contact, 74, 75
  opposite toe off, 69
  power exchanges, 74, 75, 76
  support moment contribution, 84, 85
  tibia vertical, 79
  toe off, 76
Ankle angle
  definition, 58
  gait cycle, 58, 59
  potentiometer measurement, 149
Ankle (second; mid-stance) rocker, 70
Ankle–foot orthosis, 198
Ankle-level (Syme's) amputation, 129
  amputee gait, 131, 132, 133
Antagonist, 28
Antalgic gait, 121
Anterior cruciate ligament, 9
  rupture, 188
Anterior horn, 22
Anterior pelvic tilt, excessive, 109
Anterior root, 16, 22
Anterior trunk bending, 107-8, 108, 114, 116
  above knee amputee gait, 129
Anterior, use of term, 2
Arm movements
  abnormalities, 122
  children, 94
  feet adjacent, 77
  gait cycle, 62, 63
  heel rise, 72
  initial contact, 65
  loading response, 67
  mid-stance, 70
  opposite initial contact, 74
  opposite toe off, 68
  tibia vertical, 78
  toe off, 75
Assistive devices see Walking aids

Asymmetric rhythmic disturbance, 121
Ataxia, 185
Athetosis, 122, 185, 201
Axillary crutch, 125, 125
Axon, 16, 20, 21, 22
  action potential propagation, 23, 24

B
Baclofen pump, 205, 215, 216
Balance problems see Stability problems
Balanced traction, 35, 35
Ball and socket joint, 8
Barefoot/shod gait studies, 58
Basal ganglia, 196
Base of support see Walking base
Below knee (transtibial, BK)
    amputation, 129
  amputee gait, 131-3, 132
Bertec force platform, 58, 82, 164
Biarticular muscles, 11
Biceps femoris, 13-14
  hip rotation abnormality, 114
Biomechanics, 31-45
  center of gravity, 36, 37
  circular motion, 41-2
  energy, 43-4
  force, 32-6
  historical aspects, 50
  inertia, 42
  kinematics, 42
  kinetics, 42
  linear motion, 40-1
  mass, 31-2
  moment of force, 36-40, 38
  momentum, 42
  power, 43-4
  time, 31
  work, 43-4
Body image impairment
  lateral trunk bending, 107
  spastic hemiplegia, 197
Body, lateral displacement, 91-2, 92
Body size influences, 57
Bones, 5-8, 6
Botulinum toxin injections, 215
Bounce gait, 205, 208
Bow legs, 3
Brain, 21, 22, 29, 195, 196
  damage, 25
    cerebral palsy see Cerebral palsy
    spasticity, 29, 202-3
    spinal reflexes disinhibition, 29
  motor control, 30
Brainstem motor nuclei, 196

Braking double support see Loading response
Broad based (Hemi; crab) cane, 124
'Butterfly diagram', 59, 61, 81, 163, 164

C
Cadence
  calculation, 144, 146
  elderly people, 97
  terminology, 56-7
  see also Cycle time
Calcaneus (os calcis), 7, 8
  deformity
    cerebral palsy, surgical overcorrection, 201
    excessive knee flexion, 116
    insufficient push off, 120
Calcium pump, 27
Canadian (forearm) crutch, 125, 125-6
Canes, 122-4
  broad based (Hemi; crab), 124
  gait patterns, 126
    four-point, 127, 127
    modified three-point (three-one gait), 128
    two-point, 128
  limb loading reduction, 123-4
  modifications, 124
  moment generation, 123, 124
  quad (tetrapod), 124
  stability enhancement, 123
  two versus one, 123, 124
Carbon dioxide production measurement, 157
Cartilage, 8
Cauda equina, 15
  injury, 17, 29
Caudad, use of term, 3
CD-ROM utilization, 219-22
Cell body, 16, 20, 21
Cell membrane, ionic permeability, 22
Center of gravity, 36, 37
  historical studies, 48, 49
  minimization of excursions (determinants of gait), 88-92
Center of pressure, 80, 81-2, 82, 163, 164
Central pattern generator, 30
Cephalad, use of term, 3
Cerebellar ataxia
  rhythmic gait disturbances, 121
  walking base abnormalities, 120-1
Cerebellum, 29, 196
Cerebral palsy, 20, 186, 187, 195-217
  athetosis, 214

bony deformities, 199, 210
causes, 196-7
clinical decision making, 195
deformity limitation, 215
double hemiplegia, 200
dyskinesia, 210
examination under anesthesia, 210
extrapyramidal system abnormalities, 201
foot
  deformity, 199, 205, 209, 210-11
  rotation abnormalities, 119
gait assessment, 209-14
  electromyography, 211-12
  energy expenditure, 212-13
  future developments, 213-14
  observational analysis, 211
gait patterns, 134, 204-9
  crouch gait, *201*, 201, 209
  foot function, 205
  knee function, 205-6, *206*
  scissoring, 121
  toe walking, 185
hip rotation abnormality, 113-14
history taking, 209-10
kinematic/kinetic patterns, 206-9, *207*, *208*
  double bump ankle pattern, *208*, 208
  double bump pelvic pattern, *207*, 207
  single bump pelvic pattern, *207*, 207
lever arm dysfunction, 119, 203-4, 205, 206
orthotic treatment, 198
physical examination, 210-11
primary abnormalities, 204, 205
secondary abnormalities, 196, 199, 204, 205
spastic diplegia, 199-200, 210, 214
spastic hemiplegia, 197-8, 214
spastic quadriplegia, 200, 214
spasticity, 196, *202*, 202-3, 205, 210
  botulinum toxin/phenol injections, 215
  dorsal rhizotomy, 215
  implanted baclofen pump, 215, 216
  oral medication, 215
surgical treatment, 195, 198, 209, 216
  multiple lower extremity procedures (MLEP), 214

prior gait assessment, 195
tendon transfer, 156
tertiary abnormalities, 204-5
treatment, 214-16
  goals, 214-15
  inappropriate, 214
  options, 216-17
triplegia, 200
Cervical spinal cord injury, 17
Cervical vertebrae, 15
Charge-coupled device (CCD), 141, 170
Children
  cerebral palsy *see* Cerebral palsy
  energy consumption of walking, 87
  gait development, 94-6
Cine photography, 165, 166, 168-9, 211
Circular motion, 41-2
Circumduction
  cerebral palsy, 205
  functional leg length discrepancy, 109, *111*, 111, 113
Clinical applications, 177-8
  historical aspects, 51-2
Clinical decision making, 179-84
  cerebral palsy, 195
  hypothesis formation/testing, 179-80, 183
  team approach, 179, 182
Clinical gait assessment, 177, 178-92
  aims, 179
  cerebral palsy *see* Cerebral palsy
  clinical decision making, 179-84
    team approach, 179, 182
  data interpretation, 183
  diagnosis, 180, *181*, 185
  documentation, 185-6
  examination under anesthetic, 183
  future developments, 191, 213-14
  medical litigation applications, 186
  neuromuscular/musculoskeletal disorders, 187-91
  procedure, 182-4
    flow chart, *184*
  technical requirements, 177-8
  treatment outcome evaluation, 183-4, 189-90, *190*
Clonus, 30
Club foot *see* Talipes equinovarus
Coccyx, 5
Collateral ankle ligaments, 10
Compensation, 103, 140
Computer-controlled prosthetic knee mechanism, 130
Computerized systems
  expert systems, 180, 182

footswitches, 147
force platforms output, 161, 163, 164
instrumented walkways, 147-8
kinematic data processing, 166
potentiometer electrogoniometer devices, 150
television kinematic measurements, *169*, 170-2, *171*, 182
video data recording, 141, 211
Concentric contraction, 28, 44, 158
Conductive walkways, 147
Congenital dislocation (developmental displasia) of hip, 106, *107*
Contact phase *see* Stance phase
Coronal plane, 3
Cosmesis, treatment outcome evaluation, 184
Couple, 39
Coupled foot/leg motion
  mid-stance, 70
  opposite initial contact, 74
  opposite toe off, 69
Coxa valga, 203, 206
Coxa vara, 106
Crab (broad based; Hemi) cane, 124
Crossed extensor reflex, 30
Crouch gait, *201*, 201, 209
Crutches, 122, *125*, 125-6
  axillary, 125
  forearm, 125-6
  gait patterns, 126
    four-point, *127*, 127
    modified four-point, 128
    modified three-point (three-one gait), 128
    modified two-point, 128
    three-point, *127*, 127
    two-point, 128
  gutter, 126
Cuboid, 8
Cuneiform bones, 8
Cycle time, 53, *143*, 143
  calculation, 144, 146
  children, 94, 95
  elderly people, 97
  measurement, 143, 144
    automatic, 146-8
    direct motion systems, 148
  terminology, 56-7
  visual gait analysis, 139-40
  see also General gait parameters
Cyclogram (angle-angle diagram), *149*, 149

D

Deep, use of term, 3
Degenerative arthritis, 82

Dendrite, 20, 21, 22
Depolarization, 23, 27
Dermatomes, *18*, 18
Determinants of gait
  ankle mechanism, *91*, 91
  foot mechanism, *91*, 91
  knee flexion in stance phase, *91*, 91
  lateral displacement of body, 91-2, *92*
  pelvic obliquity, *90*, 90
  pelvic rotation, *89*, 89-90
Developmental displasia (congenital dislocation) of hip, 106, *107*
Diabetic neuropathy, pressure beneath foot, 152
measurement, 189
Digitizers, 170
Direct foot pressure mapping systems, 153
Direct motion measurement systems, 148
Distal, use of term, 3
Documentation of clinical condition, 185-6
Dorsal interossei, 15
Dorsal rhizotomy, 215
Dorsal, use of term, 2
Dorsiflexion control inadequacy, 117
Dorsum, use of term, 2-3
Double hemiplegia, 200
Double legged stance *see* Double support phase
'Double pendulum' action of leg
  feet adjacent, 77
  tibia vertical, 79
  toe off, 76
Double support phase, 53, 54, 73, *103*, 103-4
  cane use, 123
  duration measurement, 147
    direct motion systems, 148
  elderly people, 97
  kinetic/potential energy transfers, 88
  lateral trunk bending, 103
  upper body movements, 62, 63
Double-float phase *see* Flight phase
Douglas bag, 157
DVD (digital video disk) equipment, 140
  kinematic measurements, 170
Dynamic equilibrium, 40
Dyskinesia, 210

E
Eccentric contraction, 28, 44, 86, 158
Efferent neurons *see* Lower motor neurons

Elbow crutch *see* Forearm crutch
Elderly people, 96-8, *97*
  cane use, 123
  gait disorders, 187-8
  see also Age-related changes
Electrocardiogram, 158
Electrogoniometers, *149*, 149-52
  flexible strain gauges, *151*, 151
  potentiometer devices, 149-51, *150*
Electromyography, 27, 154-6, 173, 179, 180, 183, 184, 191
  cerebral palsy, 206, 209, 211-12
  children, 96
  fine wire electrodes, 155-6, 182, 183
  hemiplegia, 188-9
  historical aspects, 50
  limitations, 156
  needle electrodes, 156
  surface electrodes, 155, 182
Energy
  biomechanics, 43-4
  consumption
    amputee gait, 129, 130
    cerebral palsy, 205, 206, 209, 212-13
    children, 87
    historical aspects, 50
    normal gait, 84-7
    pathological gaits, 87, 101
    per unit distance (oxygen cost), 86-7
    per unit time (oxygen consumption), 86
    treatment outcome evaluation, 184
  expenditure measurement, 84-5, 157-9
    heart rate monitoring, 158-9
    mechanical calculations, 158
    oxygen consumption, 157-8
  kinetic, 43
  metabolism for muscle contraction, 27
  potential, 43
  transfers, 50, 87-8, 89
    intersegment, 88
  usage optimization, 87
  see also Determinants of gait
Engrams, 196
Equilibrium, 40
Equinus deformity *see* Talipes equinus
Estimated external work of walking (EEWW), 158, 184
Eversion, definition, 5
Examination under anesthesia, 183
  cerebral palsy, 210

Expert systems, 180, 182
Extension, 3
Extensor digitorum brevis, 15
Extensor digitorum longus, 14
Extensor hallucis longus, 14
External (lateral) rotation, 3
External moment, 38, 39
Extrapyramidal system, 29, 203
  abnormalities in cerebral palsy, 201

F
Fascia, 8
Fascicle, 25
Fatigue, 43, 122
Feet adjacent, 53, 63, 76-8, *77*
  cerebral palsy (foot clearance), 205
Femur, 5, 6
  head, 5, 8
  neck, 5
Fibula, 6, 7
Flexible strain gauge electrogoniometers, *151*, 151
Flexion, 3
Flexor accessorius, 15
Flexor digiti minimi brevis, 15
Flexor digitorum brevis, 15
Flexor digitorum longus, 14
Flexor hallucis brevis, 15
Flexor hallucis longus, 14
Flexor withdrawal reflex, 30
Flight phase, 54
Float phase *see* Flight phase
Foot
  arches, *11*
    lateral, 11
    longitudinal, 10-11
    medial, 11
  bones, 7, *7*, *11*
  determinants of gait, *91*, 91
  disorders
    causing hip rotation abnormality, 114
    cerebral palsy, 205, 208, 210-11
    rotation abnormalities, 119, 122
    see also Foot deformities
  feet adjacent, 77-8
  heel rise, 72
  initial contact, 66
  intrinsic muscles, 15
  joints, 10
  ligaments, 10
  loading response, 67
  mid-stance, 70
  movements, *4*, 5
    gait cycle, 63
    see also Coupled foot/leg motion
  opposite initial contact, 74

opposite toe off, 69
outline, 82, *83*
placement terminology, 54-6, *55*
tibia vertical, 79
toe off, 76
Foot clearance *see* Feet adjacent
Foot contact *see* Heelstrike transient
Foot deformities
cerebral palsy, 210-11
foot contact abnormalities, 118
foot rotation abnormalities, 119
insufficient push off, 120
Foot drop
functional leg length discrepancy, 110
spastic hemiplegia, 198
steppage, *112*, 112
Foot flat (forefoot contact), 68, 94, 95
timing measurement, 146
Foot pressure measurement, 152-4
clinical applications, 189
direct pressure mapping systems, 153
force sensor systems, 153-4, *154*
glass plate examination, 153
historical aspects, 49-50
in-shoe devices, 154
Pedobarograph, 153
problems, 152
units, 152
Foot prosthesis, amputee gait, 131, *132*, 133
Foot slap, 67, 117
Footstrike *see* Heelstrike transient
Footswitches, *146*, 146-7
design, 147
Footwear, 58
corrective, 189
in-shoe pressure measurement devices, 154
wear patterns, 66, 153
Force, 32-6
free body diagrams, *35*, 35-6
moments, 36-40, *38*
resolution into components, *33*, 33, *34*
resultant determination, 33-5
parallelogram of forces, *34*, 34, 35
triangle of forces, *34*, 34-5
Force platforms, 42, 80, 81, 160-5, *161*, 179, 180, 182
corrective footwear prescription, 189
data collection, 161-2
from both feet, 162-3
data display, 163
data interpretation, *163*, 163-4

historical aspects, 49-50, 51
kinematic system combined measurements, 172-4, *173*
mounting/location, 161
two force platforms, *162*, 162
output signals, 160-1
transients measurement, 164
Force sensor systems
foot pressure measurement, 153-4, *154*
shoe-mounted, 164-5
Forceplates *see* Force platforms
Forearm crutch, *125*, 125-6
Forefoot
bones, *7*, 7, 8
contact *see* Foot flat
movements, *4*
Four-point gait, *127*, 127
modified, 128
Free body diagrams, *35*, 35-6, 50
Frequency, 31
Friction, 35, 56
utilized coefficient, 56
Frontal plane, 3
Functional leg length discrepancy *see* Leg length discrepancy

G

Gait, 47-98
amputee *see* Amputee gait
definition, 48
determinants optimizing energy usage *see* Determinants of gait
development, 50, 94-6
elderly people, 96-8, *97*
initiation, 92-3
modification, 180
normal variation, 47, 93-4
asymmetries, 58
muscle usage, 62
research, 177, 178
termination, 92-3
treadmill, 133
with walking aids, 126-8
Gait analysis
accelerometers, 159-60, 167
direct motion measurement systems, 148
electrogoniometers, *149*, 149-52, *150*, *151*
electromyography *see* Electromyography
energy consumption measurement, 84-5, 157-9
equipment, *173*, 173
force platforms *see* Force platforms
gait cycle timing, 53-4, *54*, 146-8
gait laboratory layout, *139*

general gait parameters *see* General gait parameters
gyroscopes, 160
historical aspects, 48-52
kinematic systems *see* Kinematic measurements
kinetic/kinematic combined systems, 172-4
pressure beneath foot *see* Foot pressure measurement
terminology, 52-7
visual, 48, 137-42, 211
see also Clinical gait assessment
Gait cycle, 49, 52, 57-63, 64-80
ankle angle, 58, 59
ankle/foot movements, 63
duration, 53
feet adjacent, 53, 63, 76-8, *77*
ground reaction force vector, 62
'butterfly diagram', 59, *61*, 81, 163, 164
heel rise, 53, 63, *71*, 71-3
hip
angle, 58, 59
movements, 63
initial contact, 52, 53, 63, 64-6
joint moments/powers, 58, *60*
knee
angle, 58, 59
movement, 63
leg position, 58, 59, 62
loading response, 53, 54, 62, 63, 65, 66-7
mid-stance, 53, 62, 69-71
muscle activity, 59, *61*, 62
opposite initial contact, 53, 65, *73*, 73-5
opposite toe off, 53, 67-9, *68*
sagittal plane movements, 58
stance phase, 53
swing phase, 53
terminal foot contact, 80
terminology, 52-4
tibia vertical, 53, 78-80, *79*
timing, 53-4, *54*, 146-8
footswitches, *146*, 146-7
instrumented walkways, 147-8
toe off, 53, 54, 63, *75*, 75-6
upper body movement, 62-3
Gait laboratory
equipment, *173*, 173
layout, *139*
GAITRite, 148
Gamma motor neuron, 25, 29
Gastrocnemius, 14, 72, 73
disorders
insufficient push off, 120
knee hyperextension, 115

Gemellus inferior, 12
Gemellus superior, 12
General gait parameters, *143*, 143-6, 180, 183, 184
    measurement, 143
        accelerometers, 160
        cycle time (cadence), 143, 144
        speed of walking, 143, 145
        stride length, 143, 144-5
    video recordings, 142, 145
    normal ranges, *223-4*
Genu recurvatum (knee hyperextension deformity), 114
Glass plate examination, 153
Gluteus maximus, 12, 65, 66, 67, 68, 70, 79, 182
    posterior trunk bending, 108
Gluteus medius, 12, 70, 104
Gluteus minimus, 12
Golgi organ, 30
Gracilis, 14
Gravity, 31, 32, 40
Gray matter, 15, 22
Greater trochanter, 5
Ground reaction forces, 80-3
    components, 80, *81*
    force platform measurements, 160
    gait cycle, 62
        'butterfly diagram', 59, *61*, 81, 163, 164
        heel rise, 72
        heelstrike transient, 82, *83*
        initial contact, 64-5
        loading response, 67
        mid-stance, 70, 71
        opposite initial contact, 74
        opposite toe off, 69
    shoe-mounted force sensors, 164
    toe off, 76
    treatment monitoring, 186
    'vector projection' approach, 62
Gutter crutch, *125*, 126
Gyroscopes, 160

H
H zone, 25
Habit patterns, 185
Hallux (great toe), 8
Hamstrings, 13, 65, 66, 67, 68, 70, 77, 79, 80, 182
    disorders
        cerebral palsy, 198, 199, 207
        hip hiking, 111
        hip rotation abnormality, 114
        vaulting, 113
    surgical lengthening, 211
Hansen's disease (leprosy), 189

Harris/Harris-Beath mat, 153
Head
    attitude/movement abnormalities, 122
    injury, 187
    movements
        elderly people, 98
        gait cycle, 63
Heart rate monitoring, 158-9
Heel contact *see* Heelstrike transient
Heel off *see* Heel rise
Heel rise, 53, *71*, 71-3
    amputee gait, 130
    ankle/foot, 63, 72
    ground reaction force vector, 72
    hip, 72
    knee, 72
    moments, 72-3
    powers, 72-3
    timing measurement, 146
    upper body, 71-2
Heelpad, 8
Heelstrike *see* Initial contact
Heelstrike transient (foot contact), 64, 81, 82, *83*
    abnormality, 117-18
    measurement, 159
        force platforms, 164
        kinematic, 167
    visual assessment, 144
Hemi (broad based; crab) cane, 124
Hemiparesis, 197
Hemiplegia, 18, 188, 197
    double, 200
    walking aids, 128
    see also Spastic hemiplegia
Hindfoot
    bones, *7*, 7-8
    movements, *4*
Hip, 5, *6*
    abductor weakness, 105-6, *106*
    anatomy, 8
    angle
        definition, 58
        gait cycle, 58, *59*
        potentiometer device measurement, 149
    arthritis, 105
    congenital dislocation (developmental displasia), 106, *107*
    disorders
        anterior trunk bending, 108
        cerebral palsy, 198, 199, 206, 207, 208
        hemiplegic gait, 198
        lateral trunk bending, 104-6, *105*

lumbar lordosis increase, 109
        posterior trunk bending, 108
        rotation abnormalities, 113-14
        spastic diplegia, 199
        walking base abnormalities, 121
    false joint (pseudarthrosis), 106
    feet adjacent, 77
        internal flexor moment, 78
        power exchanges, 78
    forces
        cane use, 123, *124*
        during double/single legged stance, *103*, 103-4, *104*
        heel rise, 72
        initial contact, 65, 66
        ligaments, 8
        loading response, 67
        mid-stance, 70, 71
        moments, 65, 67, 69, 71, 74, 76, 79, 180
        movements, *4*, 8, 63
            children, 94
            elderly people, 98
        muscles, 12-13
            co-contraction, 39
        opposite initial contact, 65, 74
        opposite toe off, 68, 69
        pain, 105, 106
        power exchanges, 69, 74, 76
        support moment contribution, 84, *85*
    tibia vertical, 78-9
    toe off, 76
Hip hiking, 109, 111, *112*, 113
Historical aspects, 48-52
    clinical applications, 51-2
    descriptive studies, 48-9
    force platforms, 49-50, 51
    kinematics, 49, 51
    mathematical modeling, 51
    mechanical analysis, 50
    muscle activity, 50
History taking, 179, 182
    cerebral palsy, 209-10
Horizontal plane, 3
Hydraulic prosthetic knee mechanism, 130
Hypothesis formation/testing, 179-80, 183

I
I band, 25
Idiopathic gait disorder of the elderly, 98
Idiopathic toe walking, 185
Iliacus, 12
Iliopsoas, 12, 76, 77, 78, 182, 211
    cerebral palsy, 198, 199

Ilium, 5
In-shoe pressure measurement devices, 154
Inertia, 42
Inferior, use of term, 2
Information sources, 229-32
Initial contact, 52, 53, 63, *64*, 64-6, 82, 91
  ankle/foot, 63, 66
  children, 94, 95
  ground reaction force vector, 64-5
  hemiplegic gait, 198
  hip, 65
  knee, 63, 65-6
  moments, 66
  powers, 66
  timing measurement, 146
  upper body, 65
Initial double support *see* Loading response
Initiation of gait, 92-3
Innominate bone, 5
Insertion of muscle, 12
Instrumented walkways, 147-8
Intention tremor, 122
Internal (medial) rotation, 3
Internal moment, 38, 39
Interosseous membrane, 7
Interphalangeal joints, 10
Intersegment energy transfers, 88
Intrafusal muscle fiber, 29
Inversion, definition, 5
Ipsilateral lean *see* Lateral trunk bending
Irregular rhythmic disturbance, 121
Ischium, 5
Isometric contraction, 28, 44, 85
Isotonic contraction, 28

J

Joint anatomy, 8-11
Joint angles
  cerebral palsy/spastic diplegia, 199-200, *200*
  clinical assessment, 183
  definition, 58
  electrogoniometry, *149*, 149-52
  gait cycle, 58, 59
  kinematic measurements, 165, 166, 167
  video recording measurements, 142
Joint moments, 180, 183
  estimation methods, 62
  gait cycle, 58, *60*
Joint powers, 43-4, 158, 180, 183
  gait cycle, 58, *60*

K

Kinematic measurements, 42, 165-72, 179, 182
  accuracy, 167
  active marker systems, 172
  applications, 165
  calibrated three-dimensional systems, 165, 166
  cerebral palsy, 206-9, *207*, *208*, 209
  data collection, 166
  DVD digitizers, 170
  frame rate, 166
  historical aspects, 49, 51
  measurement errors, 167
  limb marker placement, 168
  marker movement, 167-8
  photographic systems, 168-9
  precision, 167
  principles, 165-6
  resolution, 167
  single-camera systems, 165-6
  television/computer systems, *169*, 170-2, *171*
  videotape recording, 170
  walkway requirements, 139
Kinetic energy, 43
  potential energy transfer, 68, 70, 87-8
  feet adjacent, 78
Kinetic measurements, cerebral palsy, 206-9, *207*, *208*, 209
Kinetic/kinematic combined systems, 172-4, *173*
  data analysis, 173-4
Kinetics, 42
Knee, 5, 6
  anatomy, 8-9
  angle
  definition, 58
  gait cycle, 58, 59
  potentiometer device measurement, 149
  anterior cruciate ligament rupture, 188
  cerebral palsy, 205-6, *206*
    spastic diplegia, 199
  extensor weakness, 107, *108*
  feet adjacent, 77, 78
  flexion
    excessive, *116*, 116-17
    stance phase, 67, 68, 70, *91*, 91, 94
    swing phase, 76
  heel rise, 72, 73
  hyperextension, 114-16, *115*
    deformity (genu recurvatum), 114

hemiplegic/diplegic gait, 198, 200
initial contact, 65-6
ligaments, 9
loading response, 67
mid-stance, 70, 71
moments, 66, 67, 69, 71, 72, 74, 75, 76, 78, 80, 180
movements, *4*, *9*, 63
  automatic rotation ('screw home' mechanism), 9
  children, 94
  elderly people, 98
  muscles, 12-13, 14
  opposite initial contact, 74, 75
  opposite toe off, 68, 69
  power exchanges, 67, 71, 73
  prosthesis design, 129-30
  support moment contribution, 84, *85*
  tibia vertical, 79, 80
  toe off, 76
  valgus angulation, 92
    foot contact abnormalities, 118
  varus deformity, 121
Knee-jerk reflex, 29

L

Lactic acid, 27
Lateral collateral ligament, 9
Lateral condyles
  femur, 5, 6, 8
  tibia, 6, 8
Lateral (external) rotation, 3
Lateral malleolus, 7
Lateral trunk bending, 103-7
  amputee gait, 130
  associated clinical conditions, 105-6
  hip joint forces, 104-5, *105*
Lateral, use of term, 3
Leg
  bones/joints, 6
  'double pendulum' action, 76, 77, 79
  leading, 54
  motion
    direct measurement systems, 148
    historical studies, 49
  muscles, 12-13, *13*
  position during gait cycle, 58, 59, 62
  trailing, 54
Leg length discrepancy
  anatomical, 110
  functional, 109-10, 116, 117
    causes, 110
    circumduction, 109, *111*, 111

Leg length discrepancy, (cont'd)
    hemiplegic gait, 198
  knee hyperextension, 115-16
  lateral trunk bending, 107
  rhythmic gait disturbances, 121
Leprosy (Hansen's disease), 189
Lesser trochanter, 5
Lever arm, 36
  dysfunction
    cerebral palsy, 203-4, 205, 206
    foot rotation abnormalities, 119
Lift off, 77
Ligaments, 8-11, 12
  ankle, 10
  foot, 10
  hip, 8
  knee, 9
  power exchanges, 44
Ligamentum teres, 8
Light-emitting diode (LED) markers,
    172
Limp, 102
Line of gravity, 40
Linear momentum, 42
Linear motion, 40-1
Linear velocity, 167
Litigation, 186
Loading, reduction with cane use,
    123-4
Loading response, 53, 54, 62, 63, 65,
    66-7, 91
  ankle/foot, 67
  ground reaction force vector, 62,
    66, 67
  hip, 67
  knee, 63, 67
  leg position, 62
  moments, 67
  powers, 67
  upper body, 67
Lofstrand crutch see Forearm crutch
Lower motor (efferent) neurons, 16,
    22
  injury, 29
Lumbar lordosis increase, 109, 110
  cerebral palsy
    diplegic gait, 199
    hemiplegic gait, 198
Lumbar plexus, 19, 19
Lumbar spinal cord injury, 17
Lumbar vertebrae, 15
Lumbricals, 15

M
Malignant malrotation syndrome,
    204
Malingering, 185
Mass, 31-2

Mathematical modeling, 191, 213
  historical aspects, 51
Measurement unit conversions,
    225-8
Medial collateral ligament, 9
Medial condyles
  femur, 5, 6, 8
  tibia, 6, 8
Medial (internal) rotation, 3
Medial malleolus, 6
Medial, use of term, 3
Membrane potential, 22-3
Meniscus, 9
Metatarsal (toe) break, 72
Metatarsalgia, 120
Metatarsals, 7, 8
Metatarsophalangeal joints, 10
  arthritis, 120
Methods of gait analysis, 137-74
  accelerometry, 159-60, 167
  direct motion measurement, 148
  electrogoniometry, 149, 149-52
  electromyography see
      Electromyography
  energy consumption measurement,
      84-5, 157-9
  foot pressure measurement, 49-50,
      152-4, 189
  force platform measurements see
      Force platforms
  gait cycle timing, 53-4, 54, 146-8
  gait laboratory
    equipment, 173, 173
    layout, 139
  general gait parameters see General
      gait parameters
  gyroscope applications, 160
  kinematics see Kinematic
      measurements
  kinetic/kinematic combined
      systems, 172-4
  visual, 137-42, 211
Metronome, 139, 140
Mid-foot bones, 7, 7, 8
Mid-foot break, 205
Mid-stance, 53, 62, 69, 69-71
  ankle/foot, 70
  ground reaction force vector, 62,
      70, 71
  hip, 70
  knee, 70
  leg position, 62
  moments, 71
  opposite toe off, 67
  powers, 71
  upper body, 70
Mid-stance (second; ankle) rocker, 70
Mid-swing see Feet adjacent

Midtarsal joints, 10
  locking, 74
Moment of force, 36-40, 38, 39
  calculation, 36
  couples, 39
  external, 38
  internal, 39, 40
    active, 38
    passive, 38
  normalization procedure, 40
Moment of inertia, 41-2
Moment (lever) arm, 36
Moments
  feet adjacent, 78
  generation with cane use, 123,
      124
  heel rise, 72-3
  initial contact, 66
  loading response, 67
  mid-stance, 71
  opposite initial contact, 74-5
  opposite toe off, 69
  tibia vertical, 79-80
  toe off, 76
Momentum, 42
Monarticular muscles, 11
Monosynaptic reflex, 29
Motor control, 30
Motor cortex, 22, 29, 196
Motor endplates (neuromuscular
    junctions), 22, 27
Motor neurons, 21, 25, 27, 29, 195
  lower, 16, 22
  upper, 16, 22
Motor unit, 27
  recruitment, 28
Movement abnormalities, 122
'Multiflex' foot, 131
Multiple joint disease, 188
Multiple lower extremity procedures
    (MLEP), 214
Multiple sclerosis, 24, 187
Multiple-exposure photography, 165,
    168
Muscle action potential, 27
Muscle atrophy, 28-9
Muscle contraction, 25
  actin/myosin filament interactions,
      25, 26, 27
  active (internal) moment
      generation, 38
  calcium pump, 27
  clinical assessment, 183
  concentric, 28, 44, 158
  eccentric, 28, 44, 86, 158
  energy metabolism, 27
  force generation, 27-8
    active insufficiency, 27

passive insufficiency, 28
isometric, 28, 44, 85
isotonic, 28
latent period, 27
motor unit recruitment, 28
power exchanges, 43-4
reciprocal inhibition, 28
tetanus, 27, *28*
treppe, 27, *28*
twitch, 27, *28*
Muscle fatigue, 27
muscle fiber types, 28
Muscle fibers, 25
innervation, 27
intrafusal, 29
types, 28, 212
stimulation-induced alteration, 28
Muscle filaments, 25
Muscle spindle, 29, 30
Muscle tone, 30
cerebral palsy, 204, 205, 210
Muscles
acting across ankle and subtalar joints, 14-15
acting across hip and knee joints, 12-14
acting across knee and ankle joints, 14
acting only at hip joint, 12
acting only at knee joint, 14
action during gait cycle, 59, *61*, 62
historical aspects, 50
agonists, 28
anatomy, 11-15
antagonists, 28
biarticular, 11
innervation, 21, 22, 27
insertion, 12
leg, 12-13, *13*
monarticular, 11
origin, 12
physiology, 25-9
polyarticular, 11
structure, 25-7, *26*
synergists, 28
within foot, 15
Muscular dystrophy, 187, 189
Musculoskeletal disorders, clinical gait assessment, 187-91
Myelin sheath, 24
Myelinated nerves, 24-5
recovery from injury, 25
Myelodysplasia, 187
Myelomeningocele, 134
Myofibrils, 25
Myosin, 25, *26*, 27

N
Navicular, 7, 8
Neck attitude/movement abnormalities, 122
Negligence, 186
Nerve impulse, 20-1, 22, 195
pattern generators, 29
propagation, 23-4, *24*
speed of conduction, 24-5
Nerve plexus, 18
Neuroglia, 21
Neurological disorders
functional leg length discrepancy, 110
gait abnormalities, 134-5
rhythmic disturbances, 121
Neuromuscular disorders, clinical gait assessment, 187-91
Neuromuscular junctions (motor endplates), 22, 27
Neurons, 16, 20
cell bodies, 16, 20, 21
motor, 21
physiology, 20-1
resting membrane potential, 23
sensory, 21
structure, 20, *21*
Neurotransmitter, 21, 23
Newton's laws, 31
first, 31
second, 31, 35, 42, 93
third, 31, 39
Node of Ranvier, 24
Non-support phase *see* Flight phase
Normalcy Index, 174, 213
Normalization procedures, 40, 57

O
Obturator externus, 12
Obturator internus, 12
Opposite foot contact *see* Opposite initial contact
Opposite foot off *see* Opposite toe off
Opposite initial contact, 53, 65, *73*, 73-5
ankle/foot, 63, 74
ground reaction force vector, 74
hip, 74
knee, 74
moments, 74-5
powers, 74-5
upper body, 74
Opposite toe off, 53, 67-9, *68*
ankle/foot, 69
ground reaction force vector, 69
hip, 68
knee, 68
moments/powers, 69

upper body, 68
Optoelectronic techniques, 165, 166
kinematic measurements, 172
Origin of muscle, 12
Orthoses, 17-18, 183, 184
prescription, 190-1
Orthotics, 18
Osteoarthritis, 97, 114, 187, 188
hip pain, 105
Oxygen consumption, 86
cerebral palsy, 213
heart rate relationship, 158-9
measurement, 157-8, 213
Oxygen cost, 86-7, 213
Oxygen debt, 27

P
Pain
antalgic gait, 121
foot pressure measurement, 152
forefoot, 120
hip, 105, 106
lateral trunk bending, 105, 106
use of walking aids, 122, 124
Parallelogram of forces, *34*, 34, 35
Paralysis, 17-18
Paraplegia, 17
Parkinsonism, 97, 139, 187
gait abnormalities, 134-5
gait initiation, 93
Passive insufficiency, 28
Passive (internal) moment, 38
Patella, 5, 6, 9
Patellar tendon, 6, 14
Patellofemoral joint, 6, 9
Pathological gait, 101
cerebral palsy *see* Cerebral palsy
energy consumption, 87
neurological conditions, 134-5
see also Abnormal gait
Pattern generator, 29
central, 30
rhythmic gait disturbances, 121
Pectineus, 12
Pedobarograph, 153
Pedometer, 160
Pelvic obliquity, *90*, 90
Pelvic rotation, *89*, 89-90
Pelvis, 5, 6
direct motion measurement systems, 148
energy transfers, 88
heel rise, 72
initial contact, 65
mid-stance, 70
movement during gait cycle, 63
trunk movement relationship, 62-3

Pelvis, (cont'd)
  opposite initial contact, 74
  opposite toe off, 68
  tibia vertical, 78
Peripheral nerves, 21, 22
  anatomy, 18-19
  injury, 25, 29
Peroneus brevis, 14
Peroneus longus, 14
Peroneus tertius, 14
Pes calcaneus see Talipes calcaneus
Pes equinus see Talipes equinus
Pes valgus
  foot contact abnormalities, 118
  hip rotation abnormality, 114
Pes varus, hip rotation abnormality, 114
Phalanges, 8
Phenol injections, 215
Photographic techniques, 165
  kinematic measurements, 168-9
Physical examination, 179, 182
  cerebral palsy, 210-11
Physical therapy, 183, 184
Physiological cost index (PCI), 158-9, 212-13
Physiology, 19-31, 195-6
  motor control, 30
  muscles, 25-9
  nerves, 19-25
Piriformis, 12
Plantarflexion/knee extension couple, 39, 72, 115, 118, 198, 203, 205, 209
Plantar interossei, 15
Plantaris, 14
Plexus, 18
  lumbar, 19, 19
  sacral, 19, 20
Pneumatic prosthetic knee mechanism, 130
Polarized light goniometer, 152
Poliomyelitis, 29, 114
Polyarticular muscles, 11
Polysynaptic reflex, 29-30
Popliteus, 14
Posterior cruciate ligament, 9
Posterior root, 16, 22
Posterior root ganglion, 16, 22
Posterior trunk bending, 108, 109
Posterior, use of term, 2
Potential energy, 43
Potentiometer-based electrogoniometers, 149-51, 150
  limitations, 150-1
Power exchanges, 43-4
Powers

feet adjacent, 78
gait cycle, 58, 60
heel rise, 72-3
initial contact, 66
loading response, 67
mid-stance, 71
opposite initial contact, 74-5
opposite toe off, 69
tibia vertical, 79-80
toe off, 76
Pressure beneath foot measurement see Foot pressure measurement
Pressure-relieving insoles, 189
Pre-swing, 53, 54, 73, 75
Presynaptic ending, 20, 21
Primary toe strike, 118
Pronation, definition, 5
Proprioception, 22
  disorders
    rhythmic gait disturbances, 121
    walking base abnormalities, 120
Prostheses
  above knee (transfemoral, AK)
    amputation, 129-30
    knee mechanism, 130
  ankle, 131, 132, 133
  below knee (transtibial, BK)
    amputation, 131, 132
  gait assessment in evaluation/design, 190, 191
  mechanical coupling with femur, 129
Proximal, use of term, 3
Psoas major, 12
  lengthening, 198
Psychogenic gait abnormalities, 185
Pubis, 5
Pull off, 74
Push off, 73
  insufficiency, 120
Pyramidal system, 29

Q
Quad cane (tetrapod), 124
Quadratus femoris, 12
Quadriceps, 12, 14, 66, 67, 68, 69, 70, 71, 182
  disorders
    anterior trunk bending, 107
    cerebral palsy, 198, 199, 211
    hip rotation abnormality, 114
    knee flexion excess, 116
    knee hyperextension, 114, 115
    poliomyelitis-related paralysis, 114-15
  electromyography, 155
Quadriceps tendon, 6, 14
Quadriplegia, 17

R
Radian, 41
Range of motion, 139
Reach (terminal swing), 78, 79
Reciprocal gait (with walking aids) see Four-point gait
Reciprocal inhibition, 28
Recruitment of motor units, 28
Rectus femoris, 12, 72, 74, 75, 76, 77, 78
  cerebral palsy, 198, 199, 206
  surgical transfer, 211
Reference planes, 3
Refractory period, 24
Research applications, 177, 178
  technical requirements, 177
Respiratory quotient, 157
Reticular nuclei, 202
Rheumatoid arthritis, 187, 189
  lateral trunk bending, 105
  pressure beneath foot, 152
Rhythmic disturbances, 121
Rollator, 126
Roll-off phase, 73
Running, 93
  transition from walking, 54

S
SACH foot, 131
Sacral plexus, 19, 20
Sacral vertebrae, 15
Sacroiliac joint, 5
  functional leg length discrepancy, 110
Sacrum, 5
Sagittal plane, 3
  movements
    children, 94, 95
    gait cycle, 58
Sampling interval, 31
Sartorius, 13
Scalar quantities, 32
Scissoring, 121
Scoliosis, 107
Second double support see Pre-swing
Second (mid-stance; ankle) rocker, 70
Semimembranosus, 13
Semitendinosus, 13
Sensory disorders, walking base abnormalities, 120
Sensory neurons, 21, 22
Sesamoid bones, 6
Shock-attenuating footwear, 159
Shoe wear, 58
  foot pressure assessment, 153
  heel pattern, 66
Shoulder
  energy transfers, 88

gait cycle, 62
heel rise, 72
initial contact, 65
mid-stance, 70
opposite initial contact, 74
opposite toe off, 68
toe off, 75
Shuffling gait, 135
SI (Système International) units, 32
Single support (single limb stance),
    54, 73, 103-4, *104*
cane use, 123
children, 96
duration measurement, 147
elderly people, 97
energy transfers, 88
opposite toe off *see* Opposite toe off
Skin marking, 142
Slippage, 55-6
Slipped femoral epiphysis, 106
Slow walking, 140
Soleus, 14, 72, 73
insufficient push off, 120
Solid-state accelerometers, 159
Solid-state gyroscopes, 160
Spastic diplegia, 199-200
bony deformities, 210
joint angles, 199-200, *200*
Spastic hemiplegia, 197-8, 214
gait classification, 197-8
    Group I, 198
    Group II, 198
    Group III, 198
    Group IV, 198
surgical treatment, 198
Spastic quadriplegia, 200, 214
Spasticity, 30
cerebral palsy, 196, *202*, 202-3,
    205, 210, 215
dorsiflexion control inadequacy,
    117
foot contact abnormality, 118
functional consequences, 203
functional leg length discrepancy,
    110
hip rotation abnormality, 113, 114
knee flexion excess, 116
knee hyperextension, 115
stretch reflex disinhibition, 202
treatment, 205, 215
Speed of walking, *143*, 143
calculation, 145, 146
elderly people, 97
energy consumption
    per unit distance (oxygen cost),
        86-7
    per unit time (oxygen
        consumption), 86

measurement, 143, 145
direct systems, 148
normalization procedures, 57
terminology, 56-7
treatment outcome evaluation,
    184
visual gait analysis, 139, 140
see also General gait parameters
Spina bifida (myelomeningocele), 134
Spinal canal, 15
Spinal cord, *17*, 21, 22, 195, 196
anatomy, 15-18, *16*
ascending tracts, 16
descending tracts, 16
injury, 16-18, 25, 187
    cervical, 17
    lumbar, 17
    muscle atrophy, 28-9
    spinal reflexes disinhibition, 29
    thoracic, 17
motor control, 30
Spinal nerves, *17*
anatomy, 15-18
roots, 15, *16*
Spinal reflexes, 29-30
higher center inhibition, 29, 30
Spirometer, 158
Stability problems
cane use, 123
cerebral palsy, 204, 205
spastic diplegia, 199
spastic hemiplegia, 197
walking base widening, 106, 120-
    1, 130
Stamping, 118
Stance phase, 53, 54, 75
ankle, 63
duration measurement, 146
    direct motion systems, 148
energy usage optimization
    (determinants of gait), 91
functional leg lengthening, 110
ground reaction forces, 80-1
hip, 63
knee, 63, 66
    flexion, 67, 68, 70, *91*, 91, 94
subdivisions, 53
upper body, 62, 63
Stance time, 53
Starting walking, 92-3
Step factor, 57
Step length, 55, 57, 82
direct motion measurement
    systems, 148
Steppage
functional leg length discrepancy,
    109, 111-12, *112*, 113
hemiplegic gait, 198

Stiff-legged gait, cerebral palsy, 198,
    200
surgical treatment, 211
Stopping walking, 92-3
Stopwatch measurements, 143, 144
Stretch receptors, 29
Stretch reflex, 29, 30, *202*, 202
Stride length, 54, 55, 90, *143*, 143
calculation, 144-5, 146
children, 94, 95, 96
elderly people, 97, 98
height relationship, 95
measurement, 143, 144-5
    automatic, 147
    direct motion systems, 148
see also General gait parameters
Stride time *see* Cycle time
Stride width *see* Walking base
Stroboscopic illumination, 170
Stroke, 187
foot drop, 110
functional leg length discrepancy,
    110
lateral trunk bending, 107
spastic hemiplegia, 197
Subtalar (talocalcaneal) joint, 7, 8, 10
movements, 10
muscles, 14-15
Superficial, use of term, 3
Superior, use of term, 2
Supination, use of term, 5
Support moment, 84, *85*
Support phase *see* Stance phase
Surgical treatment, 183, 184
cerebral palsy, 195, 209, 216
    spastic hemiplegia, 198
Swing phase, 53-4, 57, 75, 76, 77
accelerometer/gyroscope studies,
    160
ankle, 63
children, 94, 96
duration measurement, 147
    direct motion systems, 148
functional leg shortening, 110
hip, 63, 65
knee, 65-6
    flexion, 63
subdivisions, 53
upper body, 62, 63
Swing time, 53
Syme's amputation *see* Ankle-level
    amputation
Synapse, 21, 23
Synergism, 28
Synovial joints, 8
Synovial capsule, 8
Synovial fluid, 8
Syphilis, 118

T

Tabes dorsalis, 118
Tacho-generator, 148
Talipes calcaneus (pes calcaneus), *118*
  heel loading, 117-18
Talipes equinovarus (club foot), 83, *119*
  cerebral palsy, 205
  foot contact abnormalities, 118
Talipes equinus (pes equinus), *119*
  anterior trunk bending, 108
  cerebral palsy, 205, 209
    overcorrection, 201
    spastic diplegia, 199
  foot contact abnormality, 118
Talocalcaneal joint *see* Subtalar joint
Talocrural joint *see* Ankle joint
Talus, 7
Tandem gait, 55
Tarsometatarsal joints, 10
Telephoto lens, 166
Television image analysis, 166
Television/computer kinematic systems, *169*, 170-2, *171*, 182
Temporal gait parameters *see* Gait cycle, timing
Tendons, 11-12
Tensor fascia lata, 12-13, 70
Terminal contact, 75, 80
Terminal double support *see* Pre-swing
Terminal rocker, 73, 91
  abnormalities, 118
    insufficient push off, 120
Terminal stance, 53, 70, 71, 72, 74
Terminal swing (reach), 78, 79
Termination of gait, 92-3
Terminology, 52-7
  abnormal gait, 102
  cadence, 56-7
  cycle time, 56-7
  foot placement, 54-6, 55
  gait cycle, 52-4
  speed, 56-7
Tetanus, 27, *28*
Tetraplegia, 17
Tetrapod (quad cane), 124
Thoracic spinal cord injury, 17
Thoracic vertebrae, 15
Three-one gait, 128
Three-point gait, *127*, 127, *128*
  modified (three-one gait), 128
  step-through/step-to, 127
  swing-through/swing-to, 127
Thrusting double support *see* Pre-swing

Tibia, 6, 6
Tibia vertical, 53, 78-80, *79*
  ankle/foot, 79
  'double pendulum' action of leg, 79
  hip, 78-9
  knee, 79
  moments, 79-80
  powers, 79-80
  upper body, 78
Tibial tubercle, 6
Tibialis anterior, 14, 67, 76, 79, 182
  disorders
    dorsiflexion control inadequacy, 117
    foot contact abnormality, 118
Tibialis posterior, 14, 211
Tibiofibular joint, 7
Time, units, 31
Toe clearance, 78, 79
  elderly people, 98
Toe drag, 117
Toe in, 55
  abnormalities, 113, 119
  angle, 81
Toe (metatarsal) break, 72
Toe off, 53, 54, *75*, 75-6
  ankle/foot, 63, 76
  'double pendulum' action of leg, 76
  ground reaction force vector, 76
  hip, 76
  knee, 76
  moments, 76
  powers, 76
  timing measurement, 146, 147
  upper body, 75
Toe out, 55
  abnormalities, 113, 119
  angle, 81
    elderly people, 98
    measurement, 144
Toe walking, 185
Torque *see* Moment of force
Transfemoral amputation *see* Above knee amputation
Transients measurement
  accelerometers, 159
  force platforms, 164
Transtibial amputation *see* Below knee amputation
Transverse plane, 3
Treadmill gait, 133
Treatment evaluation
  outcome, 183-4, 189-90, *190*
  progress monitoring, 186
Trendelenburg gait *see* Lateral trunk bending
Trendelenburg's sign, 105, *106*

Treppe, 27, *28*
Triangle of forces, *34*, 34-5
Triceps surae, 14, 69, 70, 71, 72, 74, 75, 76, 182
  children, 96
  disorders
    cerebral palsy, 199, 205
    dorsiflexion control inadequacy, 117
    foot contact abnormality, 118
    foot rotation abnormality, 119
    hip rotation abnormality, 114
    insufficient push off, 120
    knee hyperextension, 115
    lever arm deficiency, 119
Triplegia, 200
Tripod, 124
Trunk
  accelerometry, 160
  anterior bending *see* Anterior trunk bending
  energy transfer, 88
  feet adjacent, 77
  forward displacement measurement, 148
  gait cycle, 62, 63
  heel rise, 71
  initial contact, 65
  lateral bending *see* Lateral trunk bending
  loading response, 67
  mid-stance, 70
  opposite initial contact, 74
  opposite toe off, 68
  tibia vertical, 78
  toe off, 75
Twitch, 27, *28*
Two-point gait (with walking aids), 128
  modified, 128
Type I muscle fibers (slow twitch), 28, 212
Type II muscle fibers (fast twitch), 28, 212
Type A nerve fibers, 24
  alpha, 25
  beta, 25
  gamma, 25
Type B nerve fibers, 24, 25
Type C nerve fibers, 24, 25

U

Unmyelinated nerves, 25
Upper body
  feet adjacent, 77
  gait cycle, 62-3
  heel rise, 71-2
  initial contact, 65

loading response, 67
mid-stance, 70
opposite initial contact, 74
opposite toe off, 68
tibia vertical, 78
toe off, 75
Upper motor neurons, 16, 22
injury, 29

V

Valgus, definition, 3
Varus, definition, 3
Vastus intermedius, 14
Vastus lateralis, 14
Vastus medialis, 14
Vaulting
amputee gait, 130
cerebral palsy, 205, 214
functional leg length discrepancy,
109, 112-13, *113*
hemiplegic gait, 198
'Vector projection', 62
Vector quantities, 32, 40
Velocity, 40, 41
angular, 41, 167
Ventral, use of term, 2
Vertebrae, 15, *16*
Vestibular nuclei, 202
Vicon television/computer system, 58
Video cameras/camera-recorders, 52,
141
Video cassette recorder (VCR), 52,
141
Video recording, 140, 141, 166, 179,
180, 182, 183, 211
abnormal gait detection, 142
advantages, 140, 141
general gait parameter
measurements, 142, 145
kinematic measurements, 170
patient instruction applications,
141
skin marking, 142

teaching applications, 141
visual gait analysis, 140-2
method, 142
walkway requirements, 139
Videotape digitizers, 170
Visual gait analysis, 137-42
cerebral palsy, 211
cycle time (cadence), 139-40
gait abnormality detection, *138*,
138
gait assessment, 140
gait laboratory layout, *139*
general gait parameters
measurement, 143
historical aspects, 48
limitations, 138
video recording, 140-2
walkway length, 139

W

Waddling gait, 103, 106
see also Lateral trunk bending
Walk ratio, 57
Walkers *see* Walking frames
Walking
definition, 47-8
historical observations, 48
locomotor system requirements,
101
motor control, 30
net moment measurement, 38-9
slow, 140
speed *see* Speed of walking
starting/stopping, 92-3
transition to running, 54
Walking aids, 101, 122-8
cerebral palsy, 205, 213
spastic diplegia, 199
gait patterns, 126-8
four-point, *127*, 127
modified four-point, 128
modified three-point (three-one
gait), 128

modified two-point, 128
three-point, *127*, 127, *128*
two-point, 128
Walking base, 55, 82, 92
abnormalities, 120-1
causes, 120
children, 94, 96
elderly people, 97, 98
measurement, 144
narrow, 121
wide, 120-1
amputee gait, 130
lateral trunk bending, 106
Walking frames, 122, 126
gait patterns, 126
modified three-point (three-one
gait), 128
three-point, *127*, 127
Walking sticks *see* Canes
Walkways
conductive, 147
instrumented, 147-8
length, 139
visual gait analysis, 139
width, 139
Weakness
functional leg length discrepancy,
110
hip rotation abnormality, 113,
114
Weight, 31
Weight acceptance *see* Loading
response
Weight release *see* Pre-swing
Whip foot, 122
White matter, 15
Whole-body calorimetry, 157
Work, 43-4

Z

Z line, 25
Zimmer frame, 126